Wellness on Time
Magazine

Volume 1, Issue 1, August/September 2023

The Women
in Wellness
Edition

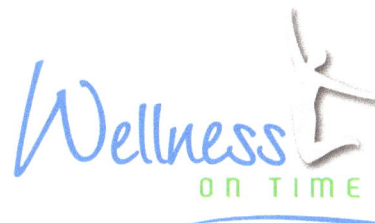

Wellness
on time

wellnessontime.net

Wellness on Time

Magazine

Volume 1, Issue 1, August/September 2023

Wellness on Time CEO, Founder, Publisher, Editor-in-Chief Natalie Pickett

Design Firestar Studios

Ad Partnerships Manager Kirsty Grace Ph +61 403 151 550 or email info@wellnessontime.com

Image credits Canva and Shutterstock. Interview features supplied their own images, and the images for the Olivia Newton John feature were supplied by the Olivia Newton-John Cancer Wellness and Research Centre. Tarot Card image on page 42 editorial by Alina Vaska/Shutterstock.com

Subscription and circulation enquiries info@wellnessontime.com

Administration and Publication Assistants Brandon Abarro and Melody Grace Lua

Wellness on Time Magazine, Volume 1, Issue 1, ISBN 978-0-6458943-0-1 is published by Wellness on Time, PO Box 1137, St Kilda South VIC 3182, Australia. +61 412 568 215. ACN 168 942 238

© Wellness on Time MMXXIII www.wellnessontime.com

From the Editor

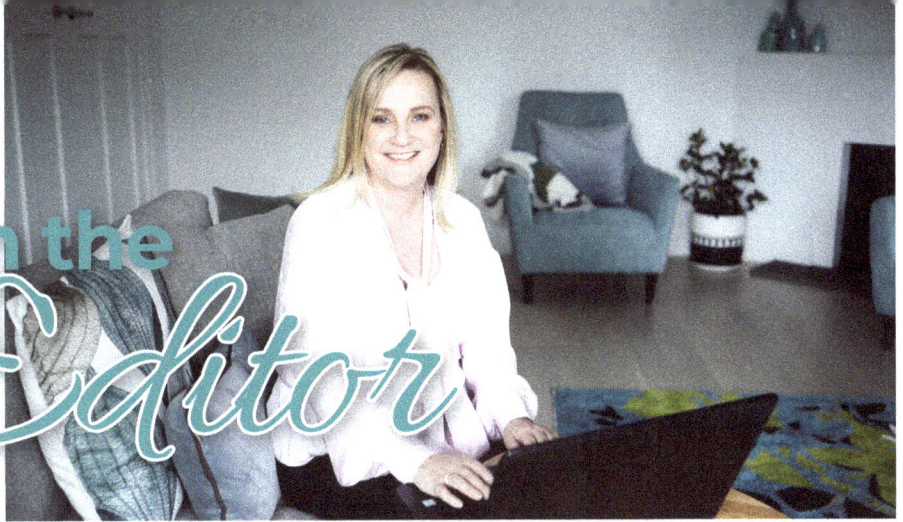

It's a pleasure to introduce you to our inaugural issue of the *Wellness on Time Magazine*. I established 'Wellness on Time' in 2014, and 'Make it easy, make it fun' is one of our mottos. It came from understanding how difficult it is to plan and include wellness activities in our daily schedules. Making time, prioritising activities, knowing what to do, fear of working out at the gym or studio with others, haven't got the right workout gear – are all reasons preventing people from getting started.

After discovering easy ways to improve wellbeing, I wanted to show others how to make it easy to integrate wellness activities into their lives. That was the impetus to start Wellness on Time as an online program with short segment activities that can be easily integrated into your day – activities that be done at home or at your desk at work, without lots of planning. This program continues today, and has evolved to be a 7-day or a 28-day program. To make it even more convenient, we now deliver your activities directly to your inbox every day.

I'm a serial entrepreneur of almost 30 years and an international best-selling author. All of my businesses and my writing comes from my passions and wanting to share knowledge with others. 'Wellness on Time' is about connecting people to quality programs and products, to assist them to easily integrate wellness into their lives. Adding magazines and book publishing is the natural extension to the online wellness concept.

I'm so excited and feel honoured to be publishing what we have included in our first issue – the Women in Wellness edition. I am grateful to everyone who has shared their wisdom. This is a global magazine with a global audience. We have women from all over the world sharing their knowledge and stories about what they do and tips for ways to improve your wellbeing.

Our feature story is about Olivia Newton John and her legacy of wellness and patient care through the Olivia Newton-John Cancer Wellness and Research Centre. Our Women in Wellness interviews feature 10 amazing women sharing their stories. We explore Shamanic wellness, charities supporting women, collaboration for holistic care, tarot for self-discovery, and spices and tips on how to boost your immunity and for integrating wellness activities. There are book reviews, a wellness wordplay, sign-up links to our programs, and links to free gifts of recipes and meditations.

Thank you for being here! We hope you enjoy everything we've included as much as we do.

Stay well!

Natalie Pickett

Entrepreneur, Speaker, Mentor

Wellness on Time Magazine

Volume 1, Issue 1, August/September 2023

In this issue ...

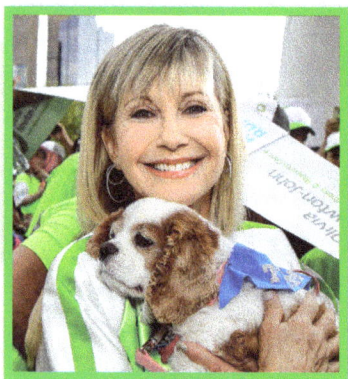
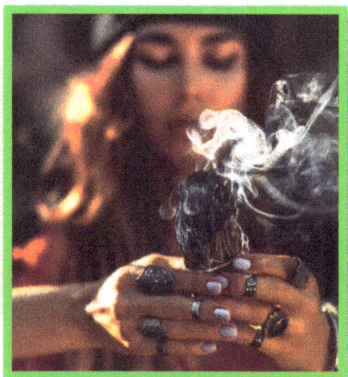

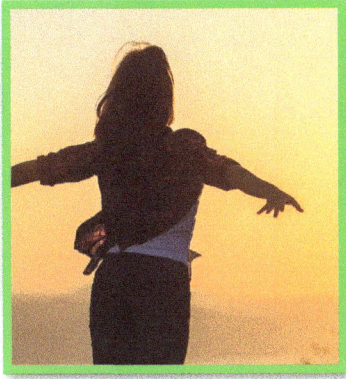

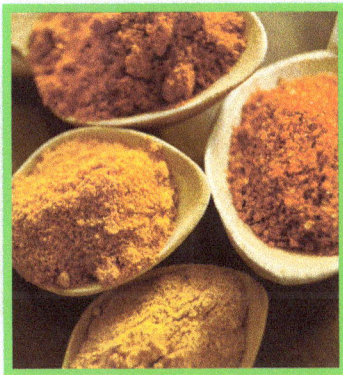

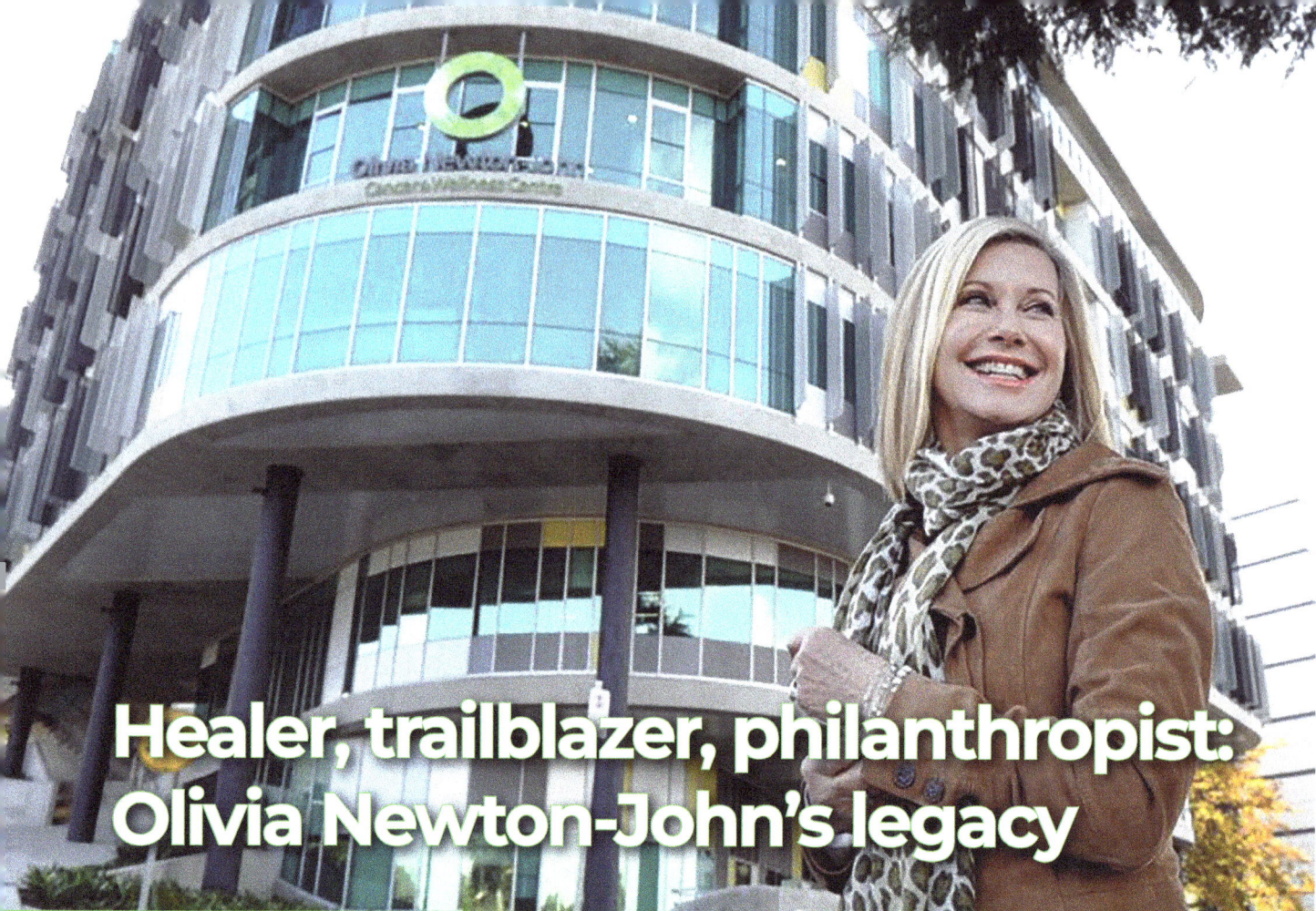

Healer, trailblazer, philanthropist: Olivia Newton-John's legacy

In an interview following the death of her beloved aunt Olivia Newton-John, Tottie Goldsmith explained that supporting people with cancer was Olivia's life work.

'It was so important to her. When people came up and wanted to talk about her career, she would always steer it back into the work she was doing for cancer,' said Tottie in the 2022 interview with *60 Minutes*.

Olivia's cancer journey

Olivia was first diagnosed with breast cancer in 1992, on the same weekend her father died of cancer. She underwent a partial mastectomy, chemotherapy, and breast reconstruction, complementing this treatment with herbal formulas and meditation to focus on a vision of complete wellness.

She was diagnosed again in 2013 after finding a lump in her shoulder. In 2017, 25 years after her first diagnosis, Olivia revealed she had been diagnosed with stage 4 breast cancer that had metastasized to her back.

'The whole experience has given me understanding and compassion, so much so that I wanted to help others going through the same journey. With more and more people affected by cancer every day, I believe we are in a world desperate for healing, and I'm committed to doing whatever I can to help,' Olivia explained.

A pioneer treating mind, body and spirit

In the early 2000s, Austin Health in Melbourne approached Olivia to help build a cancer centre. After initial hesitation, Olivia said she would only be involved if the centre embraced the concept of wellness. She wanted 'wellness' in the name, in the treatments and in every room.

The Olivia Newton-John Cancer Wellness and Research Centre (ONJ Centre) opened in 2012.

'When I was going through breast cancer in 1992, it was really important to me to have complementary wellness therapies. I thought, "Wouldn't it be amazing if a public hospital could have those same therapies for patients – the same support system I had,"' said Olivia after the ONJ Centre opened.

Olivia was a true visionary. The ONJ Centre was the first cancer hospital in Australia to combine cancer treatment and wellness programs such as mindfulness, massage, acupuncture, art therapy and music therapy, under one roof.

Wellness was fundamental in guiding not just the treatment philosophy, but also the design of the centre. It was a genuine partnership with Olivia. She worked with the

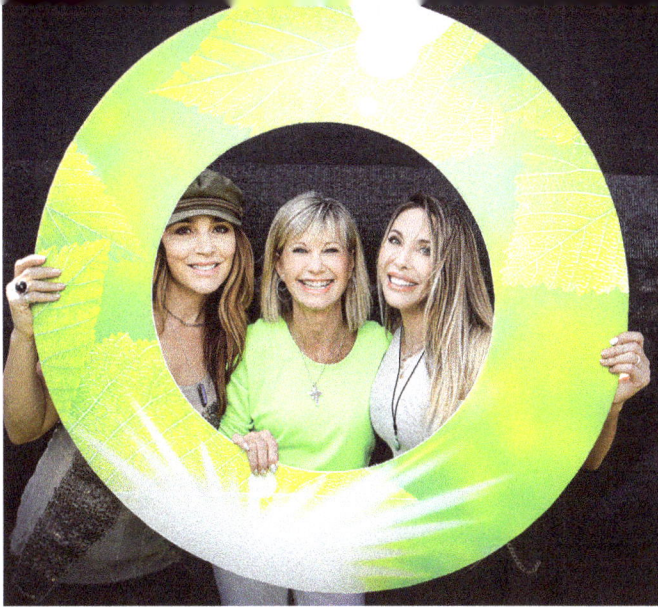

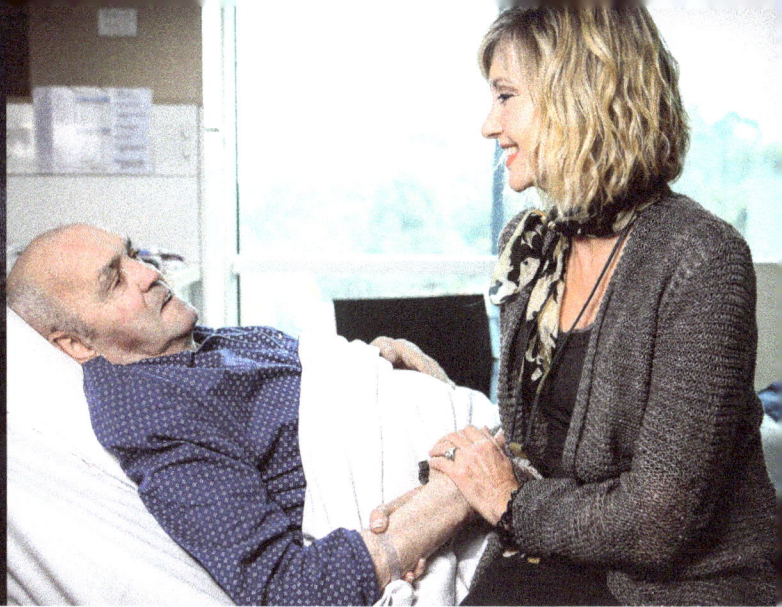

architects, influenced floorplans, and chose colours and textures. She made sure the building was filled with light, had a garden to escape to and balconies so patients could feel the fresh air.

Today, these wellness programs have been proven to reduce the pain and side effects of cancer treatment, but 20 years ago, combining wellness and cancer treatments within a public hospital was unheard of. Olivia was a pioneer. She had a groundbreaking vision to create a holistic approach to treating cancer that looked after the whole patient — mind, body, and spirit. Through the ONJ Centre, she created a place to do just that.

At the ONJ Centre today, research into many facets of cancer is untaken, as well as clinical trials and translation of the research outcomes into clinical practice. This research happens side by side with patients receiving world-class treatment and tailored wellness programs.

Olivia knew that cancer was more than just a physical journey. To truly win over cancer, you needed to support the mind and the spirit as well. The hospital is a place for treatment, and she made sure the wellness centre was a sanctuary for healing, helping patients and their families to manage their challenging experiences in the best way possible.

The power of positivity

Whenever Olivia was in Melbourne, she made it a priority to visit and talk to staff and patients at the ONJ Centre. Her ability to remain grounded and present made those private conversations very special for patients. She said that she got more out of those visits than the patients did, but it's likely patients got as much out of those visits as her.

A former staff member recalled seeing a patient the day after Olivia had met with him. 'I walked into the room not knowing what to expect – this man was very ill at the time. But he was still beaming from the day before.' Olivia left patients feeling uplifted – not because of her fame, but because of the understanding that comes from a shared human experience. Olivia was a healer.

'We hear from patients who never even met Olivia, that Olivia guides them on their journey,' said the staff member. Part of the impact Olivia had on patients was due to her own positive attitude towards life and cancer. Olivia knew being positive and feeling supported was helpful to her, and she wanted everyone to know the same support that was so important to her.

Through her long experience with cancer, Olivia remained positive and purposeful. She channelled her attitude into action, advocating for cancer research and kinder treatments, with the ultimate goal to 'see an end to cancer' in her lifetime.

> 'Cancer treatment is vital, the treatment has given me life, but the wellness programs have given me hope and to combine the two together – incredible.'
>
> Suzi, Olivia Newton-John Cancer Wellness and Research Centre patient

She was always careful to keep her language positive – saying that cancer shouldn't be a called a 'struggle' or 'battle', but simply an 'experience' in life. Olivia always signed her emails, letters and autographs 'love and light' – and ultimately her aim was to bring love and light to those with cancer.

Olivia firmly believed, 'When you go through something difficult, even something as dramatic as cancer, something positive will come of it.' And through her work supporting other patients, she realised that belief.

'My dream is that one day the ONJ Centre will be only about wellness, and we will no longer need cancer centres because cancer will be a thing of the past,' Olivia said.

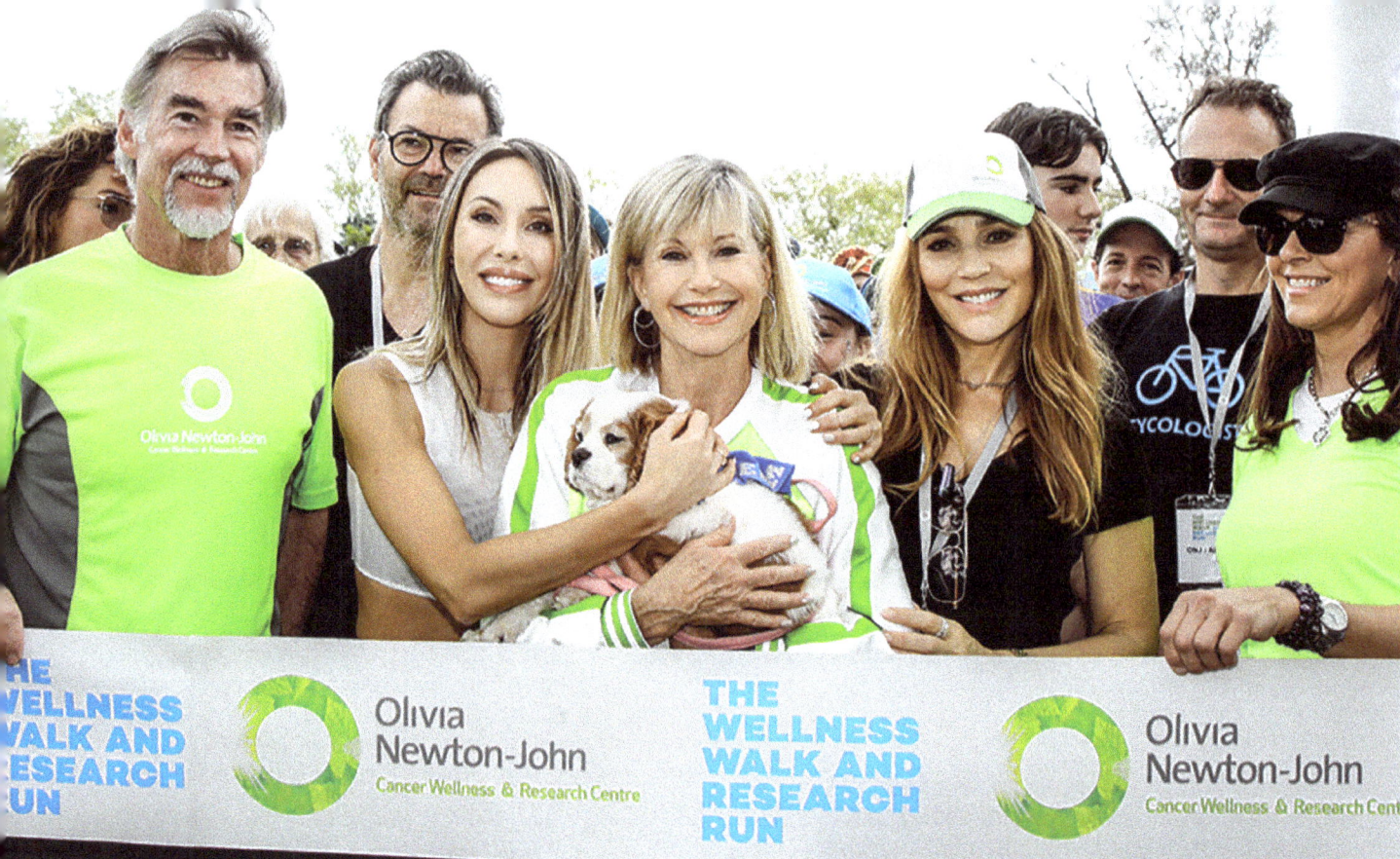

A woman of action

The wellness centre was only the beginning of Olivia's impact. For the next 20 years, Olivia led fundraising campaigns and lobbied for donations to ensure people would receive the wellness programs she knew would help. The ONJ Centre's wellness programs are not government funded, and so rely on community support to ensure they can be accessed by as many people as possible.

One of the key fundraising campaigns Olivia led was 'Olivia's Walk for Wellness', an annual charity walk that began in 2013 and continues today. Olivia invited the public to attend the walk from the shopping centre in the Melbourne suburb of Ivanhoe, to the ONJ Centre, and back, to raise money for the centre's wellness programs. Olivia said at the time, if anyone was surprised to see her walking down the suburban street, 'I am hoping they'll join me – it will be like the Pied Piper.'

Olivia's Walk for Wellness evolved into an annual event that now takes place live in Melbourne's Alexander Gardens and virtually, with walkers around the globe. It was one of Olivia's favourite events of the year, and she was said to plan her entire year around it. Each year thousands of people would join with her to fundraise to support cancer patients and raise money for wellness programs.

Continuing her legacy

Heartbreakingly, Olivia passed away in August 2022, just two months before the annual walk. Olivia's Walk for Wellness went ahead to continue her legacy of fundraising for essential wellness programs at the ONJ Centre.

A record-breaking 4,000 people came together to take part, raising more than $2.6 million to support people with cancer. The funds went to the wellness programs Olivia championed, supporting cancer patients at the ONJ to continue to thrive.

Tottie Goldsmith, ONJ Centre's Goodwill Ambassador, joined with Olivia's family and friends to lead the walk for her aunty, while Olivia's husband, John Easterling, and daughter Chloe Lattanzi, joined in from the US.

'This was one of her favourite events and favourite days because she loved seeing everyone come together to show their support for people with cancer. We could feel her love and presence with us all day', said Tottie.

Those left behind are the guardians of Olivia's vision. Her loved ones, like Chloe, Tottie and John, are dedicated to continuing to walk in her honour each year and support the ONJ Centre for the years to come.

The love and light she wished for everyone and the gratitude and hope she displayed, will forever live on through the work of the ONJ Centre and Olivia's Walk for Wellness.

Olivia's Walk for Wellness will take place on Sunday 8 October at Alexandra Gardens, Melbourne, Australia. It is also possible to participate virtually or to donate without walking. To support the walk and Olivia's vision for wellness, visit walkforwellness.com.au

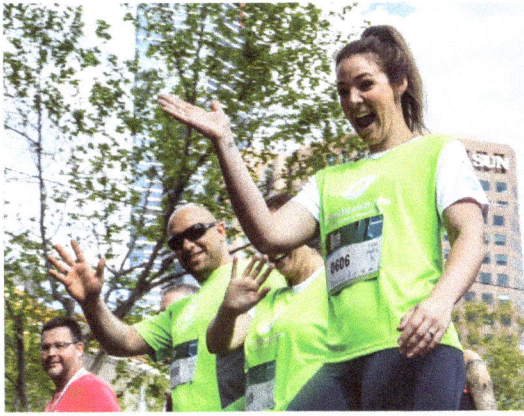

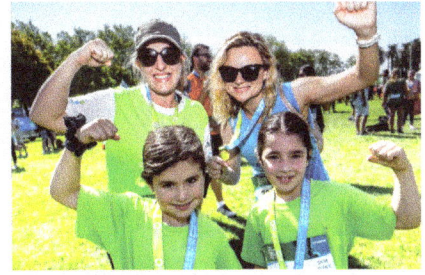

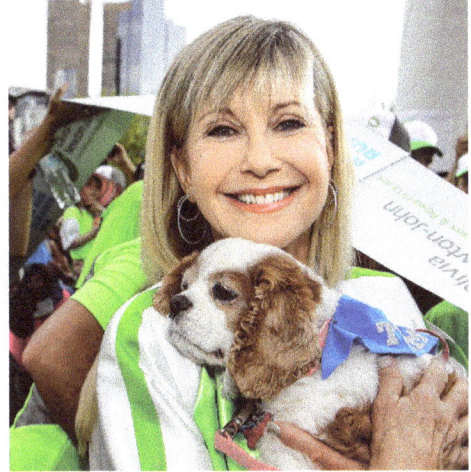

Olivia's
Walk for
♡ Wellness

Walk for Olivia and bring love & light to those with cancer

Join us live at Alexandra Gardens or virtually
Sunday 8 October 2023

Show your support and sign up to Olivia's Walk for Wellness
walkforwellness.com.au

Olivia Newton-John
Cancer Wellness & Research Centre

Austin HEALTH

'Bite-sized' wellness

by Natalie Pickett

Stress, anxiety, obesity are key health problems and causes of many diseases, some of which can be fatal. Many can be avoided by moving more and creating a healthy lifestyle. When I founded 'Wellness on Time', the program was designed with lots of short workouts that can be easily integrated into your day – activities that be done at home or at your desk at work, without lots of planning. You can click and go! It came from an understanding of how difficult it is for people to plan and include wellness activities in their daily schedule.

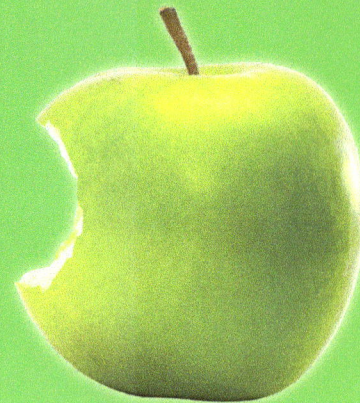

Time is a big factor, but so is not knowing what to do. You may have been told that you need to exercise for at least 30 minutes or more to get a health benefit – and when you can't find that time in one block, you end up doing nothing.

Studies show that integrating short wellness activities throughout your day will have a health benefit. Research published in *The American Journal of Health Promotion* showed that an active lifestyle that includes engaging in physical activity for less than 10 minutes multiple times a day can have the same health benefits as more structured exercise.

Additionally, researchers at Pennington Biomedical Research Center in Baton Rouge, Louisiana, studied 464 women who weren't exercisers. After six months, a group who walked an average of 72 minutes a week (just 10 minutes a day), had significantly improved heart strength and general fitness, nearly matching the efforts of women exercising almost twice as long.

'Your body responds very positively, very quickly to even small amounts of exercise,' says lead study author Tim Church, MD, PhD. 'If you're sedentary, you'll see a lot of your greatest gains going from zero to 10 minutes a day. We've seen significant changes in the autonomic nervous system – fewer incidences of the fight-or-flight stress reflex being triggered – with even 70 to 75 minutes a week of exercise. A little exercise can do much more than people think, so there's no excuse for not getting up and just doing something.'

Research has also revealed that those who sit for lengthy periods of time have twice the risk of developing diabetes, cardiovascular disease and even premature death compared to those who break up long sitting periods with regular standing or moving. Metabolism slows down 90 percent after 30 minutes of sitting. The enzymes that move the bad fat from your arteries to your muscles, where it can get burned off, slow down. The muscles in your lower body are turned off, and after two hours, good cholesterol drops 20 percent.

Even if you went to the gym for an hour in the morning then sat all day, the earlier effort is negated by the prolonged inactivity. Our bodies are designed to move. The remedy is as simple taking five-minute breaks throughout the day to get things going again.

If you discover that you have been sitting for long periods without moving it's time to change some habits. Taking breaks will not only improve your physiological wellness, but help you be more productive. Move around, go for a short walk, do some stretches at your desk.

Short workouts are time efficient – you can integrate them into your day. They increase your metabolism, improve your heart health, improve muscle toning and strength, enhance mood and energy levels, alleviate stress, and improve mental clarity and focus. Making the time, finding something you like, and remembering what to do is the key. Other studies have shown that sitting less and breathing well can slow the aging process.

People are embracing the holistic view of a wellness lifestyle. In 2021, the Global Wellness Institute identified 'wellness snacking' as a top trend. With increasing value placed on work/life balance and more remote working opportunities, the rise of regular, smaller bite-sized wellness activities and travel experiences is growing.

Let's implement the art of 'bite-sized' wellness and take a few minutes throughout the day to:

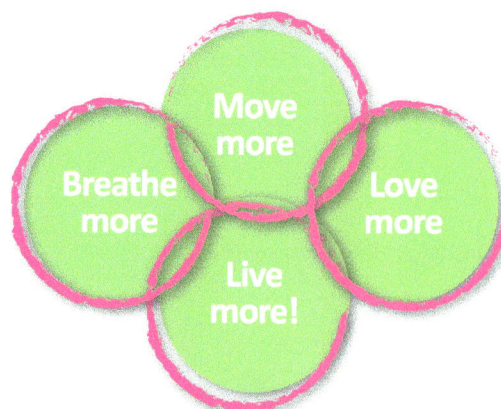

- Move more
- Breathe more
- Love more
- Live more!

You can access our 'bite-size' wellness activities in our 7 day or 28 days of wellness programs @wellnessontime

Wellness
ON TIME

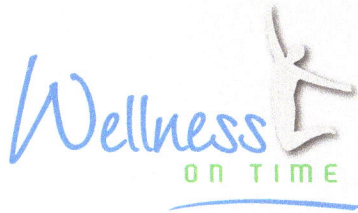

7 DAYS *of* WELLNESS

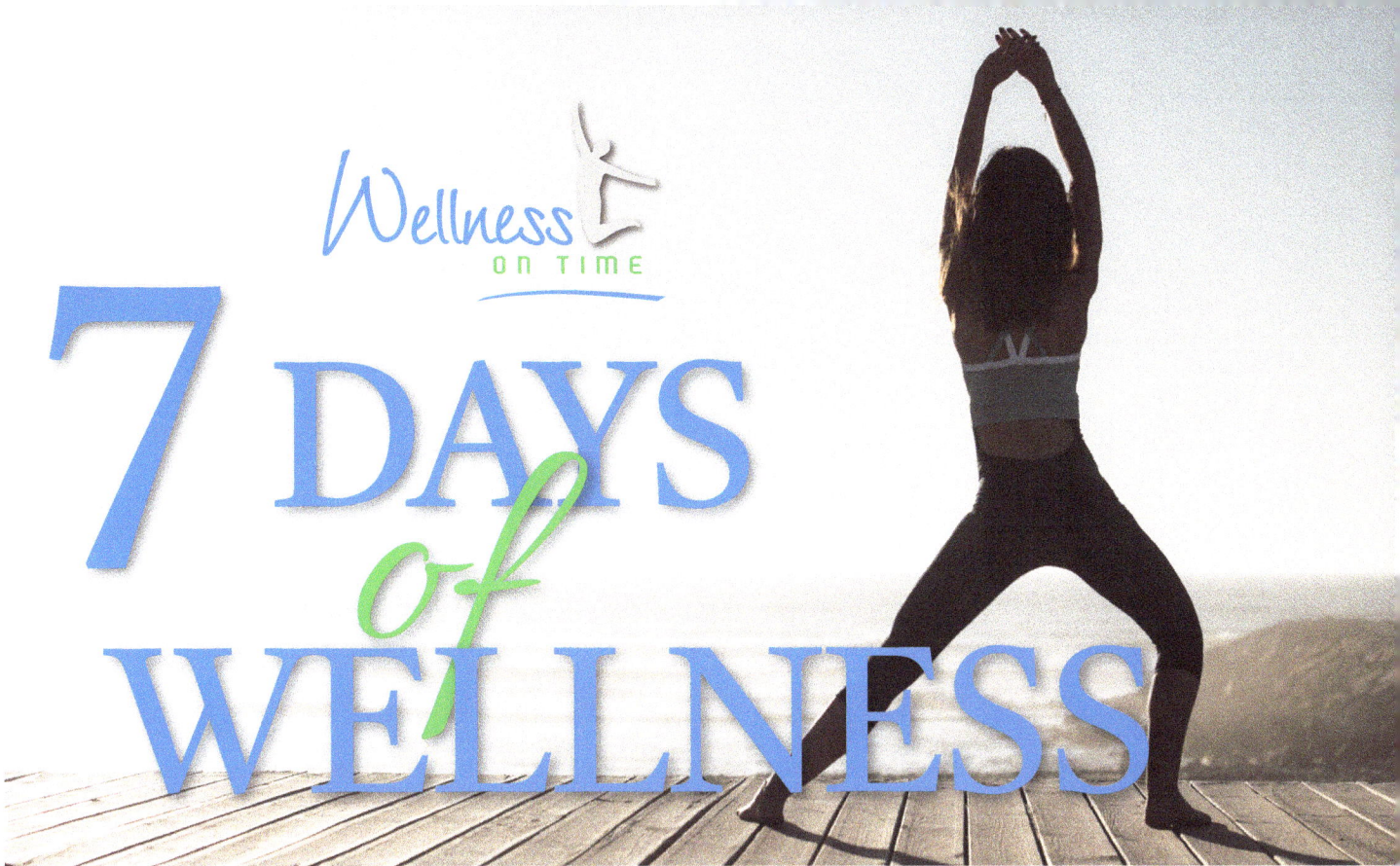

The 7 Days of Wellness program is a simple way to start integrating gentle wellness activities into your everyday.

www.wellnessontime.net/programs

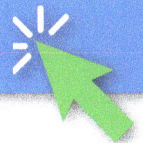

or scan our QR code

After your purchase, you will receive your email with our short video classes for the day.

Women supporting Women

When women do well, so does everyone else. Careers and businesses thrive, families and relationships are mutually supportive, and communities prosper. In the advancement of equality for women, we are very fortunate to have had strong women come before us, but there is always still more that can be done. Women around the world continue to face challenges, but support is out there. There is some amazing work happening, and we spoke with these two charities for an update on their activities.

Women for Afghan Women

Founded in 2001, Women for Afghan Women (WAW) is a grassroots civil society organisation dedicated to the right of Afghan women and girls to pursue their individual potential to self-determination, and to representation in all areas of life – political, social, cultural and economic. Prior to the Taliban takeover of Afghanistan in 2021, WAW was the largest women's rights organisation in the country, operating 32 protection centres, including women's shelters and family guidance centres, and women's rights training across the country.

The Taliban have since forced them to shutter their family guidance and women's protection centres, and many of their high-risk staff have been forced to flee the country. However, WAW remains determined to stay in Afghanistan. They have regrouped their resources, and staff have remained to respond to the dire and deteriorating humanitarian, economic and women's rights situation under the Taliban.

Today, WAW operates a Children's Support Center program that provides safe haven for 184 children whose parents are in prison or who are at risk of child marriage, abuse and trafficking. 890 staff, many of whom are women working from home due to Taliban bans, implement other programs that have distributed emergency and humanitarian aid to over 1 million Afghans (including 676,525 women and girls). Schools and clinics have been refurbished, and safe environments with counseling, training, and aid to combat gender-based violence in vulnerable communities have been created.

In the United States, WAW operates centres in New York and Virginia that are a lifeline for the immigrant communities they serve, including newly arrived Afghan refugees who benefit from resettlement support and a comprehensive network of programs. Both centres offer culturally competent domestic violence and other forms of case management, empowerment classes, legal and immigration services, and women's circles.

Despite all the challenges WAW have faced in the last two years, they continue to rise beyond crisis and look to the future with hope.

For more information and to donate visit https://womenforafghanwomen.org

Dress for Success

Dress for Success is a global not-for-profit that empowers women to achieve economic independence. With affiliates in 143 cities across 23 countries, Dress for Success has assisted over 1.3 million women globally since 1997. Dress for Success Sydney clients receive donated work clothing, and access to career support programs, coaching, and job preparation services at no cost.

In Australia, Dress for Success Sydney has supported over 17,000 women since 2009. With regional showrooms in Illawarra and Newcastle-Hunter, and affiliates now in Melbourne, Brisbane, Perth, Adelaide, and Hobart, more than 73,000 women have been supported nationwide.

Clients come from a range of backgrounds. They include young women at risk of disengaging from education, struggling single mothers, older women lacking financial security, women exiting correctional services, domestic violence survivors, women with disabilities, and newly arrived migrants, asylum seekers, and refugees. Referrals come from employment agencies, service providers, social workers, charities, and community groups.

Dress for Success Sydney aims to be the leading organisation in Australia for the empowerment of women through employability services. However, without consistent government funding, they rely on donations from fundraising campaigns and revenue from pre-loved pop-up fashion sales.

Dress for Success Sydney's programs and services are available to any woman and non-binary person in New South Wales seeking to enter or re-enter the workforce. They offer in-person and virtual styling and presentation skills, along with a range of workshops and one-on-one services such as resumé reviews, mock interviews, and mentoring.

Programs like Style Delivered and the national DFS Career Hub support women in need wherever they are (https://dfscareerhub.org.au).

To access Dress for Success Sydney's services or to donate, visit https://sydney.dressforsuccess.org. For more information about their global services visit https://dressforsuccess.org

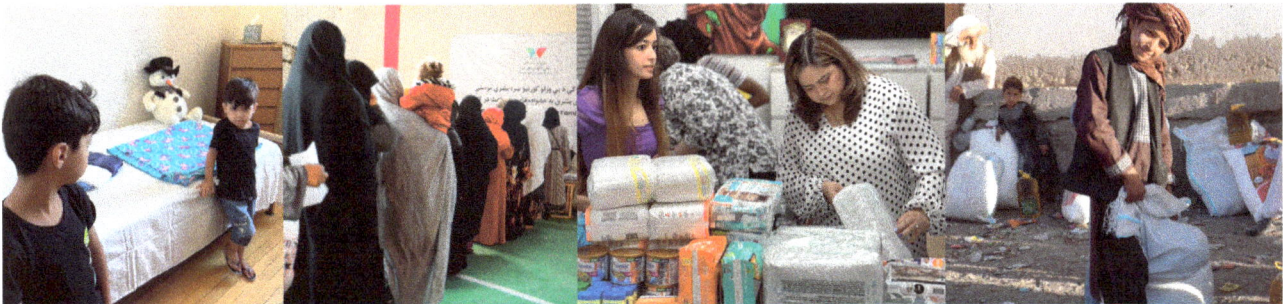

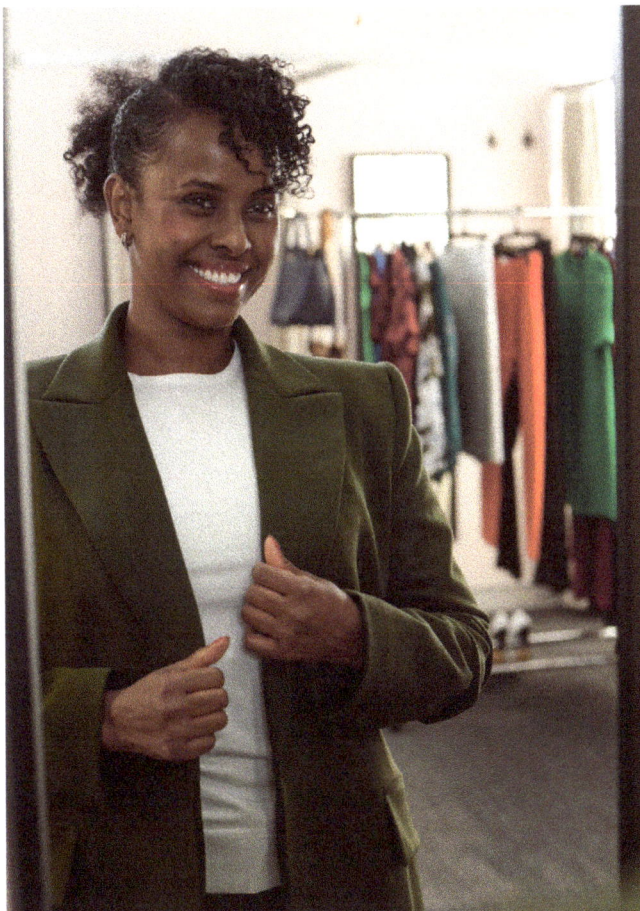

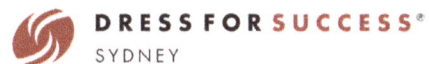

Collaborative healing teams: bridging the gap between traditional and holistic medicine

By Faryl Moore

Can you hear that? The quiet yet constant low hum reverberating through our healthcare system? What's missing? Why are people still suffering? It is time to explore what many cultures have understood for centuries – everything is energy, including disease, which means looking towards alternative approaches to work alongside traditional healthcare.

According to the National Center for Complementary and Integrative Health (NCCIH), approximately 38% of adults in the United States use some form of complementary and alternative medicine (CAM), including holistic healthcare.

Creating collaborative healing teams allows for the modern medical approach and the holistic approach to work together to provide a more comprehensive overall treatment plan for the patients. It's important to understand the benefits of a collaborative healing teams and strategies for implementing one effectively.

What is holistic healthcare?

Holistic healthcare is an inclusive approach that recognises the interconnectedness of various aspects of an individual's health. Rather than focusing solely on the symptoms of the disease, it considers the whole person. Perhaps Deepak Chopra says it best, 'In holistic healthcare, the goal is not just to treat the disease, but to restore balance and overall wellbeing.' This approach considers the idea that physical ailments are influenced by emotional, mental, and spiritual factors, and vice versa.

What are the benefits of a collaborative healing team?

1. Treats the root cause: traditional medical treatments often focus on managing symptoms rather than addressing the underlying cause of illness. By including a holistic practitioner, the collective team can identify and treat the root cause of health issues, leading to long-term healing and prevention of recurring problems.

2. Improved patient and provider relationship: healthcare providers who adopt a holistic team approach can build stronger relationships with their patients. Taking the time to listen to their patient's concerns, understand their unique circumstances, and involve them in decision making processes leads to more patient-centered care.

3. Integration of modalities: a holistic approach encourages the integration of various healthcare modalities. A survey conducted by the American Hospital Association found that 42% of hospitals in the United States are already offering one or more alternative therapies, such as acupuncture, massage therapy, or meditation as part of their healthcare services. This integration allows for a broader range of treatment options, tailored to individual needs and preferences.

4. Patient empowerment: holistic care empowers patients to take an active role in their healing process. By considering their physical, emotional, and spiritual needs, patients are more likely to feel heard, respected, and supported in their healthcare journey. This sense of empowerment can lead to increased engagement and better treatment outcomes.

Strategies for implementing a collaborative healing team

1. Communication and collaboration: effective communication and collaboration among healthcare professionals are essential for implementing an effective healing team. This includes interdisciplinary teamwork, sharing information, and actively involving patients in decision making processes. This communication needs to be a two-way street.

2. Continuous education: holistic care recognises that physical health is deeply intertwined with emotional, mental, and spiritual wellbeing. By addressing these interconnected aspects, patients often experience improved overall wellbeing, leading to a higher quality of life. Therefore, healthcare providers should pursue basic training and education on a variety of holistic modalities, enabling them to integrate complementary therapies and understand the importance of addressing the whole person in their practice. It is also important for healthcare providers to stay updated on any new modalities that are showing promise in the healing arts.

3. Creating supportive environments: healthcare settings must foster environments that support holistic care. This may involve offering integrative services, providing resources for self-care, and promoting a patient-centered approach throughout their care. It is also important for the space to feel warm and inviting, promote wellbeing, and reduce stress. Items like fluorescent lighting, and eggshell-colored walls should be replaced with lamps, and light blues, and other calming colors. Patients need to feel relaxed when they are entering care spaces.

> A holistic approach to care recognises that health is not solely determined by physical factors but also influenced by emotional, mental, and spiritual aspects.

A holistic approach to care recognises that health is not solely determined by physical factors but also influenced by emotional, mental, and spiritual aspects. By embracing this comprehensive perspective, healthcare providers can offer more personalised and effective care, leading to improved patient outcomes and overall wellbeing. As the significance of holistic healthcare continues to grow, it is crucial for healthcare systems to prioritise and integrate this approach into their practices, ultimately benefiting patients and providers alike.

Faryl Moore is the founder of Moore Energy – providing energetic care for optimum wellbeing and holistic success.

Exploring the Shamanic Priestess: ancient traditions in the modern world

By Rev. Patricia Ferreira

After my divorce, my world shattered, and the familiar embrace of the church began to slip away. The community that had once uplifted me now closed its doors, deeming me unfit to serve as an usher in the mass and support the women's retreats that had brought me much fulfillment.

This was a painful time when I yearned for God's words and acceptance, but instead, I found myself pushed to the margins. I decided to leave the church and take God with me. Little did I know that this would be the start of my journey into shamanism. Each day, my bond with the Divine grew stronger and more intimate. I discovered a direct connection to God that transcended the confines of religious institutions.

The essence and mission of the Shaman

The Shaman holds no dogma – the mission is to restore balance and harmony. They aid individuals to heal, find a deep sense of belonging and connect with their purpose by aligning them with all our relations on earth – our self, the elements, plant and animal beings. They act as intermediaries between the physical and spiritual realms. They navigate the unseen realms to seek medicine, wisdom, and guidance for themselves and their communities.

Origins and historical significance of shamanism

Shamanism is an ancient spiritual path for awakening, healing, and divination. The origins of shamanism can be traced to the earliest human societies, where individuals with innate healing abilities and a deep connection to the natural world emerged as shamans. Archaeological evidence suggests that shamanic practices were the oldest spiritual traditions known to humankind.

Shamans have traditionally existed in Indigenous cultures such as Siberia, Africa, the Americas, and Asia. However, shamanic practices are not confined to these cultures alone. In recent times, the knowledge and wisdom of shamanism have gained popularity worldwide, transcending cultural boundaries and attracting individuals seeking a deeper understanding of themselves and the Universe.

Women's role in shamanism

The history of shamanism reveals that women played significant roles as shamans, healers, and spiritual leaders in many ancient cultures. In fact, the earliest known evidence of shamanic practice found by archeologists, dating from more than 30,000 years ago, indicated that the shaman was a woman. The earliest known shamans were women who held vital positions of power and influence within their communities. Their ability to bridge the realms of the seen and unseen, their nurturing qualities, and their connection to the cycles of nature made them natural conduits for spiritual wisdom.

In retelling the stories of these early shamans, we honor the sacred feminine and acknowledge the valuable contributions of women in the spiritual realm. By embracing the priestess and shamanic practices, we reclaim the ancient wisdom that lies within our collective memory and reawaken the power of the divine feminine in the modern world.

Shamanic priestess work

Priestesses, like shamans in ancient communities, observed and honored the natural rhythms and patterns of the earth. They performed sacred rituals in alignment with the seasons, revering women as embodiments of the Great Mother and celebrating their ability to nurture life within them, much like the earth itself. Throughout history, Roman, Greek, and Egyptian priestesses inhabited holy temples, worshipping and serving the spiritual needs of their communities. However, as time passed, fear and misunderstanding grew, and the power of priestesses became viewed as a threat. Countless priestesses were persecuted, and many were forced into hiding to preserve their spiritual practices. Today, in a time marked by patriarchal dominance, a modern-day priestess is emerging, bringing forth ancient wisdom and integrating it with contemporary influences. Her mission is to awaken the dormant Divine Feminine energy and restore a harmonious balance between the masculine and feminine as a sacred union.

The modern-day application of shamanism

In today's fast-paced world, the ancient wisdom of shamanism continues to resonate with people seeking spiritual and personal growth. Shamanic healing ceremonies, visualisation, soul retrievals, and plant medicine journeys are a few examples of the techniques employed in modern-day shamanic practices.

As a shamanic priestess, I have woven the paths of shamanism and priestess to create a holistic approach to spirituality and healing. Participants connect deeply with their inner selves, the natural world, and the divine by incorporating shamanic rituals, breathwork, energy work, timeline travel, and ancient wisdom teachings into my retreats.

Shamanic priestess retreats and immersions

In my retreats, I create a sacred space where individuals can embark on their personal quests. Through shamanic journeying, participants explore their inner landscapes, confront and heal past wounds, and rediscover their innate wisdom. By incorporating shamanic priestess practices, such as ritualistic dance, sacred breathwork journeys, and devotional offerings, the retreats become transformative experiences, connecting participants to the deep well of their spirituality.

Conclusion

As the ancient ways merge with the present, shamanic priestesses offer a sacred space for seekers to embark on their own spiritual quests, harmonising the wisdom of the past with the current realities while embracing the infinite possibilities of the future. Retreats and healing journeys become transformative experiences, where individuals can find personal direction, healing, and a profound connection with the Divine.

Bibliography

https://www.rosemaryandyew.co.uk/shamanic-priestess-work/
https://www.gaia.com/article/how-much-do-you-know-about-shamanism
https://www.gaia.com/article/subtle-art-shamanism-and-energy-healing
https://insights.taylorandfrancis.com/social-justice/recognizing-the-importance-of-women-healers/
https://www.cuyamungueinstitute.com/articles-and-news/woman-shaman-the-suppressed-history

Rev. Patricia Ferreira is a Shamanic Priestess, Intuitive Success Catalyst and Author at Awakened Boss Lady Success Circle.

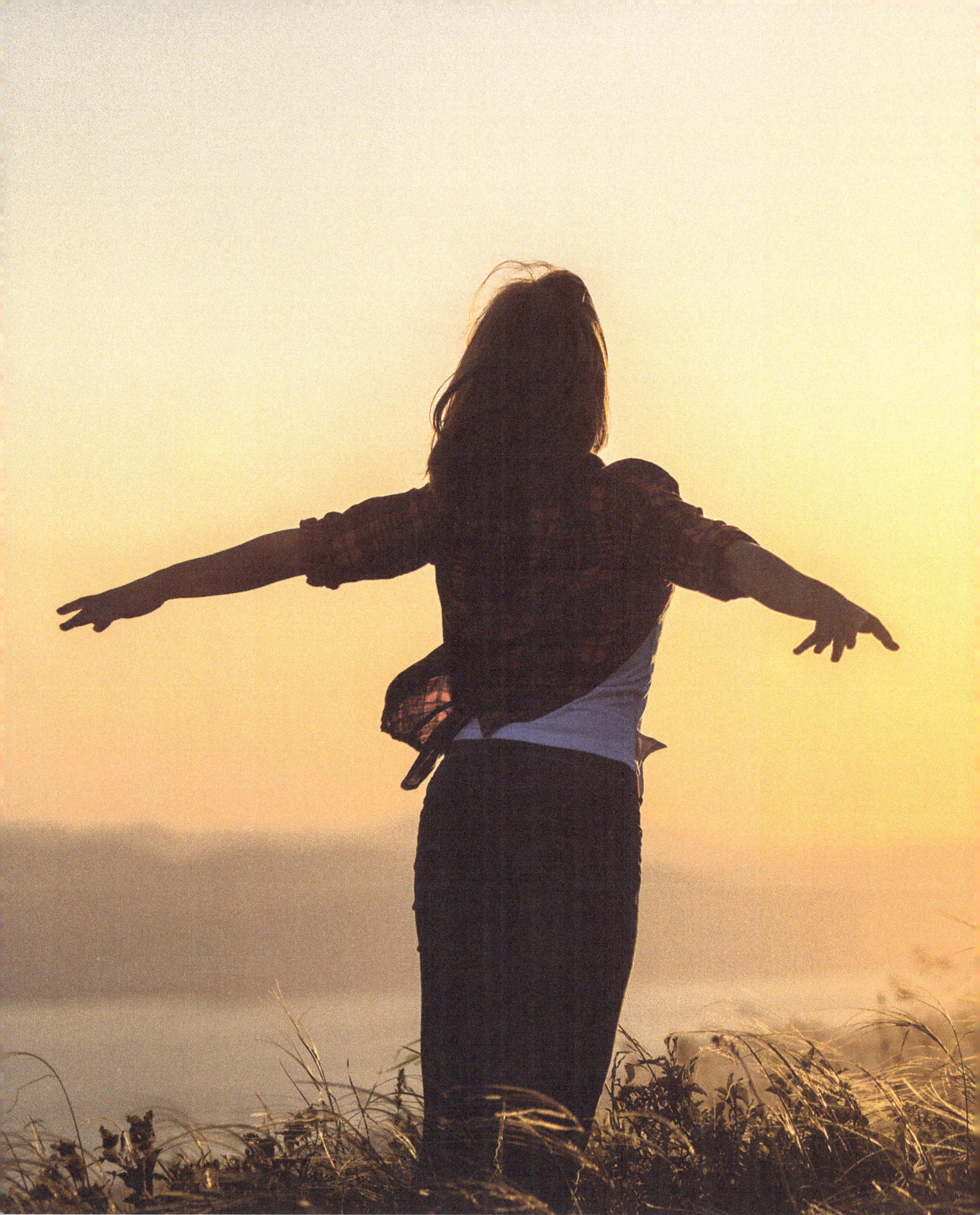

Women in Wellness

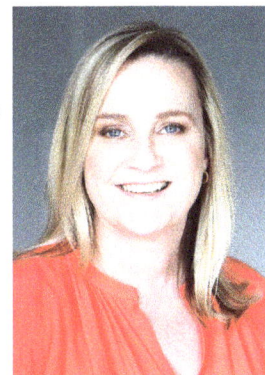

Women have made significant contributions to the wellness industry and have played a crucial role in shaping its many aspects. Is it different for women in wellness careers? Conventional medicine is often seen as a practice that treats the symptom, but not holistic in the way that it searches to identify the cause. It is also considered a male dominated domain, where women's roles have historically been associated with nurturing roles within families and broader social contexts.

Throughout history, there are examples of women not being credited for their work in medical discoveries or not taken seriously when seeking help for medical conditions, yet across cultures and timelines, women have played pioneering roles as healers and caregivers. They have served as the original healers, using their knowledge of herbal remedies, intuitive practices, and nurturing care to support the wellbeing of individuals and communities.

Women have been at the forefront of promoting and advocating for wellness in diverse ways.

As a former fitness instructor, I felt that I was already living a wellness lifestyle. It was an injury that led me to study and gain a fitness qualification. We've probably all experienced times when we have health or injury issues. When I do, I find activities that benefit my recovery to allow less need for ongoing medical intervention and greater ease of body movement. After discovering ways to heal and improve wellbeing, I felt I had found answers that I wanted to share. I wanted to show others how to make it easy to integrate wellness activities into their lives, and that was the impetus to start 'Wellness on Time'.

It's a common thread – these lived experiences in seeking treatment or discovering solutions that drives people to create their careers in wellness. These are the women who are influencing the wellness industry through their chosen practices.

It is an honour bringing this series of interviews from around the globe with women who have followed their passions, sought to find answers, and wanted to share their knowledge to help others.

Thank you to these amazing women for trusting us with your stories and allowing us to share them with the world.

— Natalie Pickett, Wellness on Time CEO, Founder, Publisher, Editor-in-Chief

Melanie Gleeson

endota CEO

Can you tell us a bit about your background? Has wellness always been an important focus for you?

I was raised by a strong family and community who instilled a sense of inner belief and confidence that I could do anything I put my mind to. I have always seen the value in pursuing wellness and mindful practices, drawing inspiration from those around me and the natural environment.

At the age of 26, I was brave enough to take a risk and follow a dream. I opened one of the first day spas in Australia on the Mornington Peninsula, at a time when few people even knew what a spa was and fewer recognised the importance of investing in wellbeing. Today endota has 110 spas globally and is Australia's leading spa network.

I am humbled by the growth of the endota brand and feel so blessed to be doing what I love, and have people walk away after a treatment, physically and emotionally replenished.

Can you remember when you first realised that the wellness activity that you practice was an important part of your life? Was there an 'Aha!' moment like you'd solved a life puzzle?

I was working in a day spa, and the motivation for me to start my own business came from the change I saw in people once they'd had a treatment. They would come in all stressed, and their shoulders would be up near their ears – and after the treatment, they would leave an entirely different person. The physical change was so powerful. From there I thought, 'I really want to provide this feeling to more people.' I wanted to be able to make people feel better, and I wanted to be able to do it my way.

How did you get started in this area, what was the impetus to start doing what you do as a career choice? What sort of training/qualification did you need?

It was hard to sell-in the brand at first, so there was a lot of networking and education required to make it work. Once our franchisee model was well established, our biggest challenge was ensuring that every spa presented an accurate reflection of the endota brand.

Today we have an amazing network of business owners. They are our ambassadors, and they care about our clients. To ensure that every spa is an accurate reflection of the brand, we support our franchisees with training, workshops, events, and an open-door approach to communication. Our therapists are enthusiastic and engaged and choose to work with us for the same reason I started endota spa, to help people feel better.

Tell us a bit about you, where you are located, and what is the work that you do as a woman working in the wellness industry?

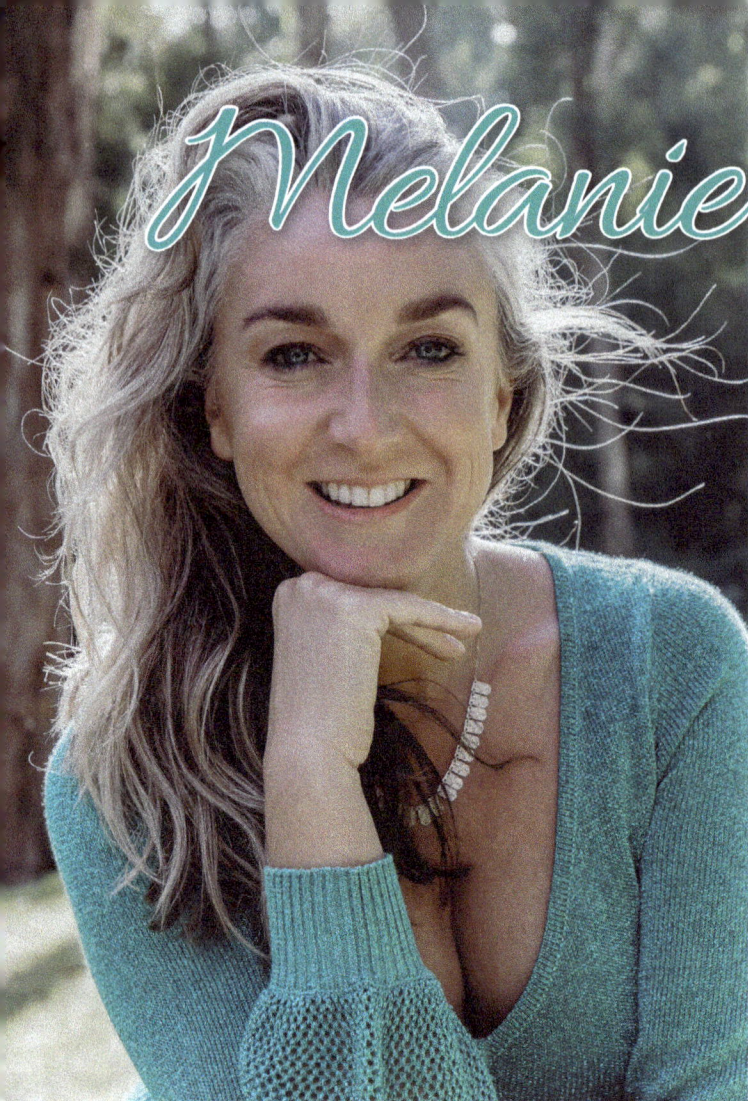

I'm Melanie Gleeson, and I live on the Mornington Peninsula in Victoria.

The endota story began in 2000, and it was inspired by the belief that something special happens when we actively nurture our health and happiness. We feel more uplifted, more confident, and more authentically ourselves, and I wanted to harness that, and see where I could take it in my community.

When I started endota, a group of female friends and I discussed what our true values were in life, and it had me thinking about what the foundation of my business would be built on. That's where I landed on Intent, Connect, Truth and Balance. Our spa, skincare and wellness products, retreat and Wellness College are all underpinned by these values as well as an approach to life and work by each employee. By offering a diverse range of wellness experiences, endota supports women on their journey towards a greater sense of wellbeing – to help them nourish and nurture the mind, body, and skin.

The evolution of endota saw us open our training school, endota Wellness College in 2018, which has been recognised for its excellence in education and commitment to high-quality training, offering nationally recognised training in Beauty Therapy, Remedial Massage and Salon Management. With campuses in Victoria, New South Wales and Queensland, our college offers flexible learning options and the opportunity to gain practical experience. endota Wellness College courses keep pace with fast-moving beauty and wellness trends, techniques, and technology, producing highly skilled beauty and wellness professionals, who are industry leaders in the field.

Do you think there is a difference for how women are treated when they are seeking help for ailments, and is it there a difference for women working in the wellness industry that brings some advantage/disadvantage?

Wellness should be seen as a necessity and not a luxury. It is so important for wellness to be integrated into our lives and not seen as an 'add on' to our traditional routines. It is all about living better, healthier, and happier and incorporating tools holistically to do so. This not only prevents sickness and physical ailments, but nurtures and nourishes our mind and spirit.

As women, we're used to wearing so many different hats – mother, wife, friend, employee. To find balance,

> It's important to find moments of small self-care that enable us to sustain a natural state of being.

it's important to take a few moments each day to reflect and practice being still. This is how I feel most connected to myself. I also believe practicing mindfulness every day is vital to maintaining a happy and balanced life. A lot of the inspiration for endota's nourish.nurture.you rebrand focuses on how it's not just about how we look, but more importantly about how we feel. If we are healthy, happy, and confident in who we are, we will feel well.

Who inspires you in the wellness industry?

Our people inspire me every day! I genuinely love the connections that I've built over 20 years in this business. I am constantly inspired by the endota staff, therapists and business owners who demonstrate a passion for wellness and making people feel better. I learn from the people in the business and I am in awe of the work they do.

Our people are good listeners, empathetic and approach building relationships in an open and honest way. These values are what I built the endota brand on, and having a team that is visibly emblematic of those values has had a huge impact on the endota story and the brand's impact on the wellness industry.

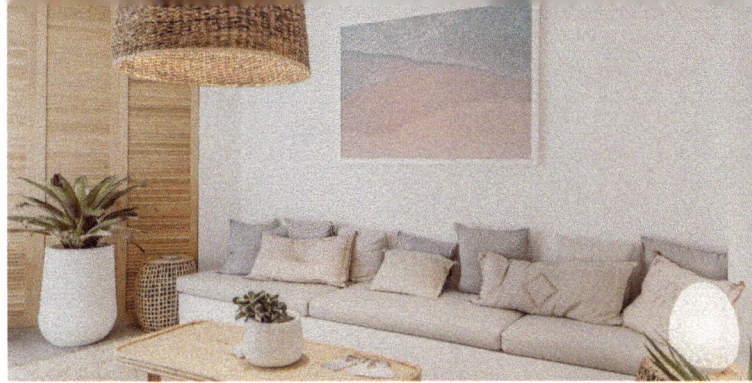

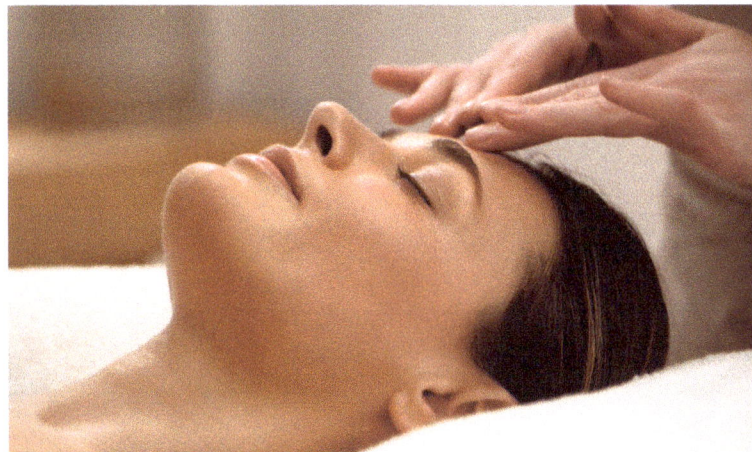

Can you provide some tips for our readers on how they can integrate wellness activities into their daily lives?

The pursuit of wellbeing is a way of life, focusing on micro-rituals that you can incorporate into your day-to-day life will help you to feel good in the moment and more resilient in the long-term.

We all juggle so much as mothers, employees and more, that we can't always take a lot of time for ourselves. It's important to be realistic and find moments of small self-care that enable us to sustain a natural state of being. Even just five minutes to sit, breathe and be present can make an impact.

Our wellness choices can enrich our minds and energise our bodies, whether that be through time in nature, taking part in meditation, Pilates, or regular spa treatments.

If you were to describe how you feel about what it means to you to be sharing your love of wellness in three words, what would they be?

Grateful, passionate and elated.

Explore ...

🌐 endotaspa.com.au

📷 www.instagram.com/endotaspa

Can you remember when you first realised that the wellness activity that you practice was an important part of your life? Was there an 'Aha!' moment like you'd solved a life puzzle?

Living by my values has always been part of me. I trained in Acceptance and Commitment Therapy (ACT) and discovered that values/work is one of the cornerstones of ACT. It was an enlightening moment for me to realise that the way I've been leading my life has been condensed in a comprehensive framework – a framework that was flexible, easy to grasp and could be transmitted to others. It felt like an incredible 'Aha!' moment, as I felt that my life experience was being empirically validated!

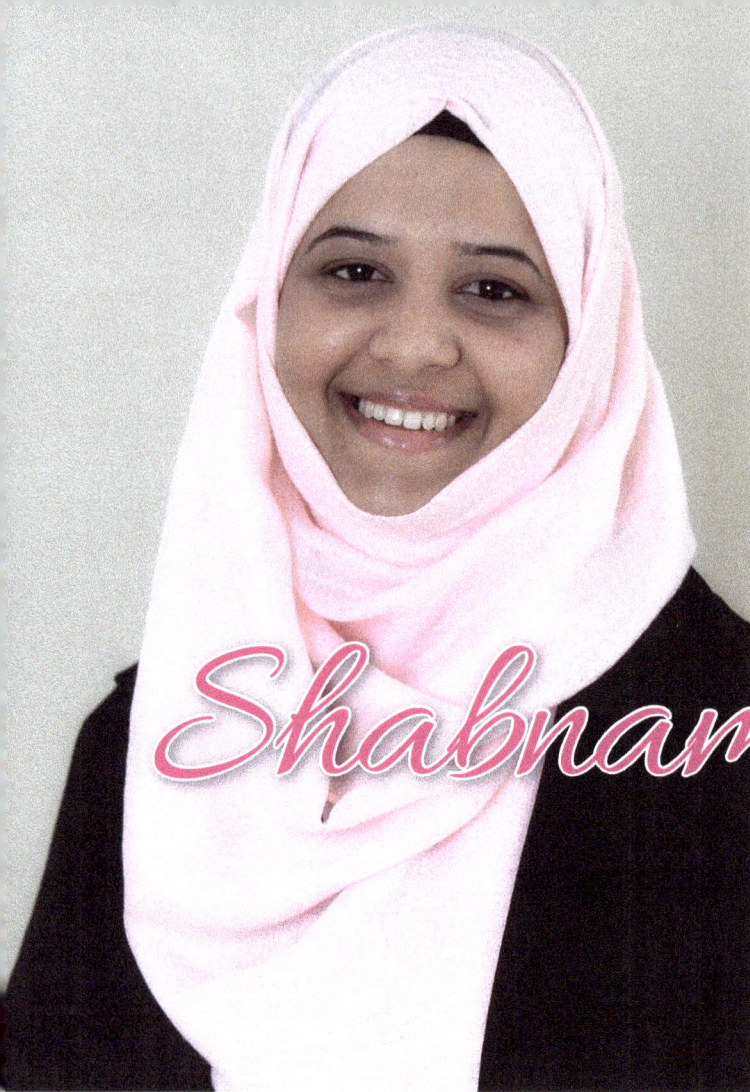

Shabnam Rakhiba

Life Coach and Chronic Illness Mentor, Thorns and Roses Coaching

Tell us a bit about you, where you are located, and what is the work that you do as a woman working in the wellness industry?

I was born in Mauritius and spent 13 years in Bermuda, after which I moved to southwest London where I currently reside with my husband and my three children.

I am a life coach and a chronic illness mentor. I support women living with chronic health conditions. I help them develop the emotional resilience and flexibility they need so they can thrive despite their illnesses.

Can you tell us a bit about your background? Has wellness always been an important focus for you?

I did not give much thought to wellness until I became unwell in my early twenties. It started with a niggling ache in my lower back that eventually spread to encompass my whole body. It's only recently, after more than 10 years, that I was diagnosed with fibromyalgia.

The years I spent undiagnosed were the hardest as chronic pain is invisible, and it felt impossible to convey the extent of the suffering to those around me. The chronic pain took a toll on my mental health, and it took years to get back to the light through therapy and life coaching.

How did you get started in this area, what was the impetus to start doing what you do as a career choice? What sort of training/qualification did you need?

I was quite confused regarding my future career path after I completed my Master in Psychology. It was difficult to investigate being employed due to the unpredictable nature of the pain I live with.

I had spent a year during my Masters exploring the experiences of women living with chronic illness. I wanted to further this exploration. I also felt called to using my lived experience with illness to guide others, so they could find ease as they navigate the difficulties that come with living with illness. I therefore trained as a CPCAB Life Coach and as an ACT practitioner and focused my practice on supporting women with health conditions.

Do you think there is a difference for how women are treated when they are seeking help for ailments, and is it there a difference for women working in the wellness industry that brings some advantage/disadvantage?

I feel that women are less likely to be taken seriously when seeking support. This week only, I've interacted with two women – one who was struggling to put in place an appropriate care plan as she has been severely disabled by long-COVID, and another who is a cancer survivor and struggling to access adequate financial help.

I have noted that many women experience a downward mental health spiral in the aftermath of interactions with unsupportive healthcare professionals. Some give up on seeking the support they deserve for fear of facing more negative judgments. Being in the wellness industry has equipped me with the emotional resilience to navigate the aftermath of difficult interactions. I feel more empowered to self-advocate and insist on the right care.

Who inspires you in the wellness industry?

Russ Harris, therapist, renowned ACT trainer and author of multiple ACT books, who I trained with briefly. One of his sayings has served me well: "Develop the courage to solve those problems that can be solved, the serenity to accept those problems that can't be solved, and the wisdom to know the difference."

Learning to let go of trying to solve problems that have no resolutions has brought peace into my life.

Can you provide some tips for our readers on how they can integrate wellness activities into their daily lives?

Here are three suggestions drawn from ACT:

1. **Stay aware** – embrace the power of now. In each moment lies an opportunity for self-discovery and healing.

    Cultivate 'present moment awareness' to fully engage with your experiences and connect with your body and mind in the here and now. As you engage in wellness activities, such as meditation or self-care practices, be fully present and observe without judgment.

2. **Stay engaged** – choose to embrace life's offerings and let your passions be your guiding light.

    Actively participate in activities that bring you joy, and fulfillment. Engaging in wellness activities can provide a sense of meaning and connection to what truly matters to you. Find activities that align with your values and engage wholeheartedly.

3. **Stay open** – in the face of challenges, let go of rigidity and flow with the winds of change. Your resilience lies in your ability to adapt.

    Chronic illness often brings unpredictability, but practicing acceptance and openness can help you adapt and find new pathways to wellness. Be open to exploring different approaches, seeking support, and adjusting your self-care routines based on your current needs.

If you were to describe how you feel about what it means to you to be sharing your love of wellness in three words, what would they be?

Passionate, purposeful, fulfilled.

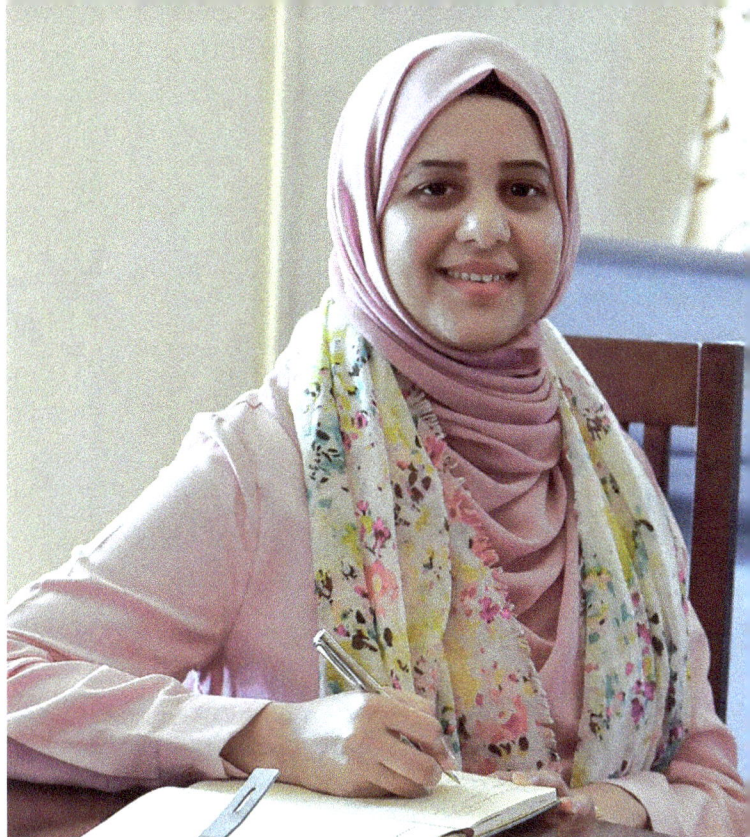

Is there anything else you would like to share with our readers?

When it comes to wellness, I believe that social connectedness plays a vital role in enhancing wellbeing. Maintaining strong social connections allows us to share our experiences, express our emotions, and receive empathy and understanding from others. During challenging times, such as living with a chronic illness, having a network of supportive individuals can help alleviate feelings of isolation and distress. Being part of a community or social group provides us with a feeling of being accepted, valued, and understood and helps foster a positive self-image. Social connectedness also has a direct impact on our physical health and has been linked to lower rates of chronic diseases, improved immune function, and increased longevity.

As a chronic illness mentor, I emphasise the importance of social connectedness and encourage individuals to seek out supportive communities, engage in social activities, and nurture relationships that contribute to their overall wellness.

Explore ...

🌐 www.thornsandrosescoaching.com

🌐 www.chronicwellnesslounge.com

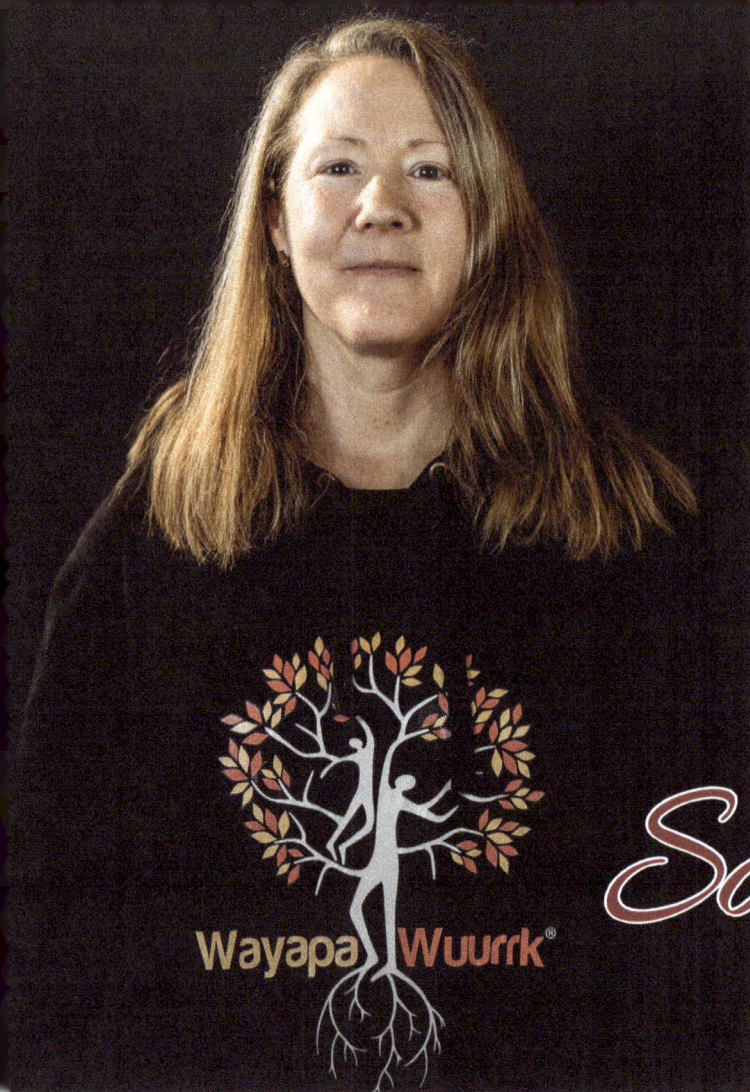

While Jamie is at the forefront sharing his Indigenous wisdom and connection to country, I am the woman wuurrking behind the scenes of our wellness business, which includes almost 300 trained Wayapa Wuurrk practitioners throughout Australia, the US, Canada, and the UK.

Can you tell us a bit about your background? Has wellness always been an important focus for you?

For my first 45 years, numbing myself was the priority in my life. From a young age, alcohol was my go-to for suppressing childhood trauma – an entrenched feeling of not fitting in anywhere and a deep void inside myself that seemed endless. But alcohol, combined with low self-esteem, led to very poor relationship choices starting a cycle of abuse that took a long time to break free from.

Although I started on my spiritual journey about 30 years ago with the discovery of meditation, it wasn't until I was gifted Wayapa 10 years ago that I understood the meaning of true wellbeing.

Sara Jones

Co-founder and Executive Director, Wayapa Wuurrk

Tell us a bit about you, where you are located, and what is the work that you do as a woman working in the wellness industry?

I was born and raised in Canada until I was 14, but my ancestry is Welsh, with both my parents having been born in Wales. They immigrated to Canada on their honeymoon and then decided to move again, this time swapping hemispheres! I have lived in Australia for 40 years, now living on the lands of the Gunaikurnai People of far East Gippsland, Victoria. I share my ancestry because it is part of understanding my connection to who I am.

I am the Co-founder of 'Wayapa Wuurrk' with Jamie Thomas, a Gunaikurnai man and Maara descendant. Wayapa Wuurrk means to Connect to the Earth in the language of the Peek Whuurrung and Gunaikurnai peoples, respectively.

Wayapa Wuurrk is a globally certified earth connection wellness modality based on the wisdom of Indigenous and ancient peoples, which focuses on taking care of the earth as the starting point for holistic wellbeing. Combining earth mindfulness and reciprocity, narrative meditation, sharing story and a physical, embodiment practice, Wayapa creates earth mind body spirit wellness.

Can you remember when you first realised that the wellness activity that you practice was an important part of your life? Was there an 'Aha!' moment like you'd solved a life puzzle?

Wayapa transformed my life, and I remember the exact moment when this missing piece of my jigsaw puzzle dropped into my life very unexpectedly, but with beautiful synchronicity, as it was something I had been calling out spiritually for my entire life. Jamie and I were talking about how I could support him to start a cultural mentoring foundation when I steered the topic to finding something that we could do to generate income for the foundation. Jamie said he had a connection practice he would sometimes share in kindergartens and schools, so he showed me for the first time what would soon be known as Wayapa Wuurrk.

After Jamie demonstrated the movement practice that he had organically cultivated for a decade, I was left speechless, receiving a massive cellular download of ancestral knowing. This was my 'Aha!' moment, as I realised the deep void inside of me that seemed like it could never be filled was the disconnection of my relationship with Mother Earth. In that instant, I knew this practice of earth reconnection needed to be shared with the world to help others just like me, so I spent the next 12 months creating a framework around it so it could be certified by the International Institute for Complementary Therapists.

How did you get started in this area, what was the impetus to start doing what you do as a career choice? What sort of training/qualification did you need?

It was the instantaneous and deep knowing that Wayapa Wuurrk needed to be shared with the world to help others who were like me, feeling such disconnection from the earth, that started me on my soul's purpose of co-creating this modality into existence. I would say I had a lifetime of training to get me to that moment of knowing – a lifetime of experiential learning of how disconnection can manifest in all sorts of self-sabotaging, unwell ways. A decade of learning to listen to the richness of Indigenous ways and trusting in the Ancestors who had guided Jamie and myself into this beautiful, heart-based creation.

Do you think there is a difference for how women are treated when they are seeking help for ailments, and is it there a difference for women working in the wellness industry that brings some advantage/disadvantage?

Of our almost 300 certified Wayapa Wuurrk practitioners, most are women because they are drawn to sharing the purpose-driven, heart-space wellness practices that resonate for them individually. Being a Wayapa practitioner also provides a flexible income stream that can be tailored to meet their own needs – whether it be wuurrking around caring for kids and family or nurturing passion projects. With a focus also on caring for the earth, creating intergenerational wellbeing and being strengths-based, Wayapa is appealing for many women.

Who inspires you in the wellness industry?

Louise Hay is my original inspiration, because she followed her passion for sharing wellbeing on her own terms, and with a thirst for lifelong learning and pioneering new ways of approaching wellbeing.

I always acknowledge and honour the Indigenous ways of knowing, being and doing that have been shared with me by Jamie, many amazing Elders, and 'deadly' First Nations people who continuously show the greatest strength, resilience, and wisdom. But ultimately, it is the jaw-dropping genius and beauty of Mother Earth that inspires me to get up every day to wuurrk to the best of my abilities.

Can you provide some tips for our readers on how they can integrate wellness activities into their daily lives?

This is a time of remembering. Remembering we are nature, that we're not separate from it, so co-create the environment that will keep you and the next generation well. Hug a tree. Not only do we have a reciprocal

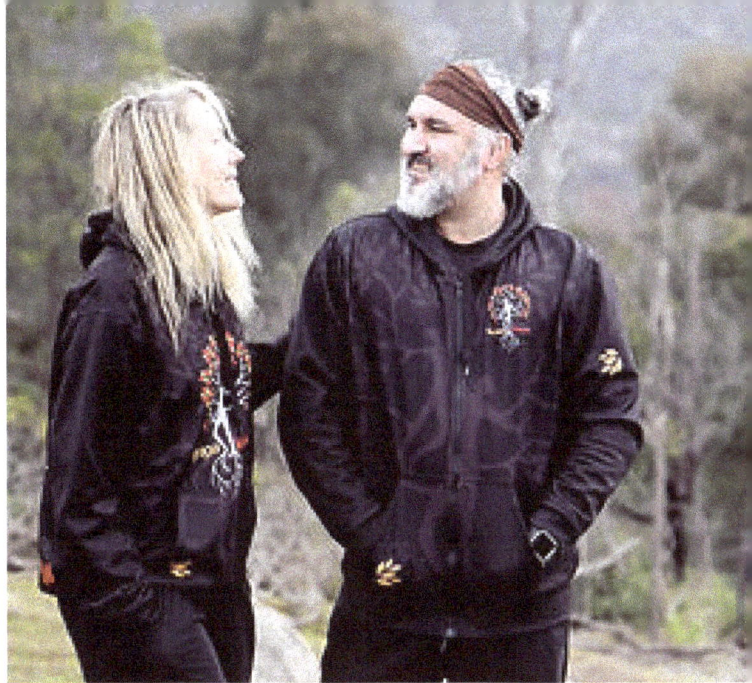

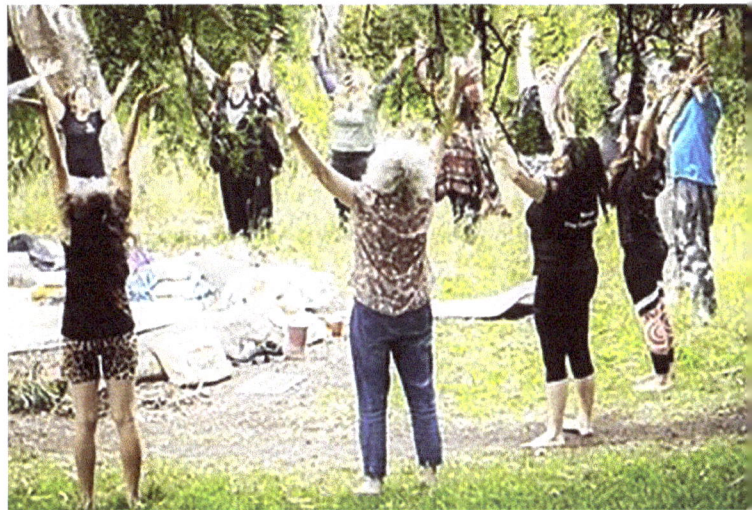

relationship with trees because they breathe out what we breathe in, they are great listeners. Hugging a tree in gratitude it makes us, and the tree, feel good.

Make time every day to connect to your environment to observe everything it provides. Watch the sun rise to give us light and warmth. Stick your tongue out in the rain to taste the water that provides life to everything. Be in flow with the moon cycles to recharge and rest. Be Wayapa.

If you were to describe how you feel about what it means to you to be sharing your love of wellness in three words, what would they be?

Giving is receiving.

Explore ...

www.wayapa.com

work, and I began to draw the body constantly. My parents even bought me a five-feet, five-inch-tall skeleton so I could learn every bone.

In college, I started studying sports medicine/athletic training, and during a kinesiology class, the professor played videos of various sports movement patterns asking us to name what muscles were firing in order for the action to happen. Because I had been drawing the body for over four years, I was able to connect the dots quickly. As an intern for my college's women's basketball team, I was able to apply what I knew about how muscles worked, where they connected, and where they inserted to determine how correcting muscle imbalances would lead to less pain and help prevent further injury.

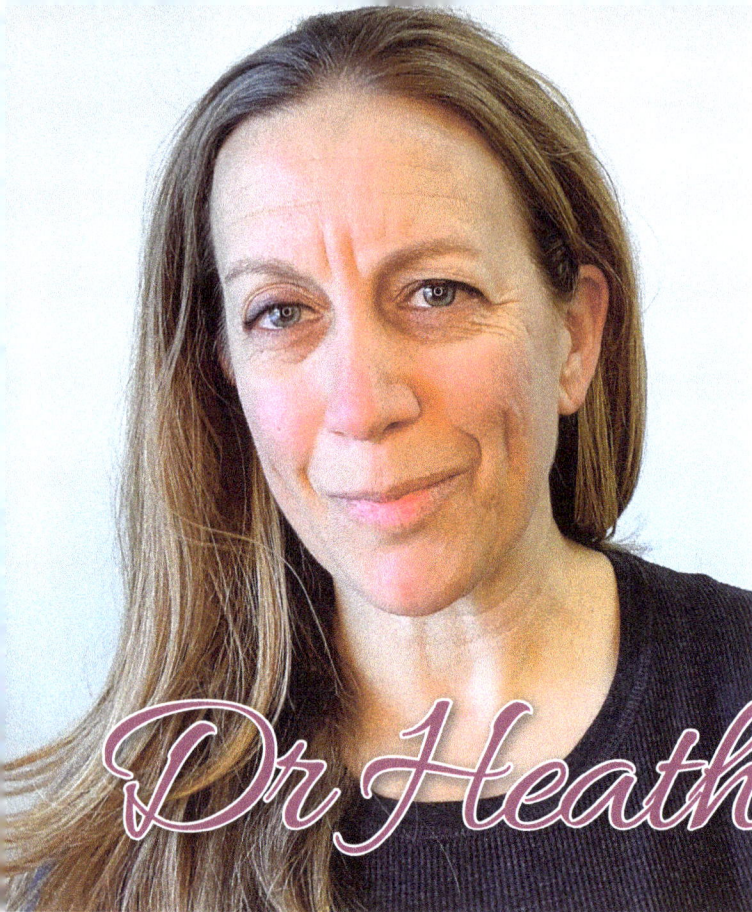

Dr Heather Gansel

Sports Chiropractor, Ask Doctor Heather

Tell us a bit about you, where you are located, and what is the work that you do as a woman working in the wellness industry?

For 22 years I have been a sports chiropractor practicing in Connecticut where I am originally from. I help athletes and non-athletes achieve optimal performance by teaching them how to fix their pain naturally through corrective exercise and rehabilitation techniques they can do from the comfort of their home.

Can you tell us a bit about your background? Has wellness always been an important focus for you?

From the age of five, I was always playing sport, and with every sport I played, I could feel the demands they made on my body. That's why it wasn't surprising when I experienced extreme pain when I was the catcher for our traveling softball team. I was 14, and fear was an automatic response because I did not know any better. I wasn't sure I would be able to walk again thanks to the massive amount of radiating pain into my legs.

Can you remember when you first realised that the wellness activity that you practice was an important part of your life? Was there an 'Aha!' moment like you'd solved a life puzzle?

It was thanks to my mother's chiropractor who utilised kinesiology (muscle testing) to determine the root cause of the problem. I became pain-free in a short period of time, and I was amazed! I was intrigued about how our bodies

How did you get started in this area, what was the impetus to start doing what you do as a career choice? What sort of training/qualification did you need?

I always wanted to be a sports chiropractor. When I was in eighth grade, I shadowed a chiropractor for Career Day, watching him give hope to patients who expressed frustration, sadness and/or pure desperation. I knew at that moment I was meant to be a healer.

In the early 1990s, sports medicine was not a common career path. Many colleges did not have it as a major, so my choices were limited. I wanted the four-year degree in sports medicine/athletic training, before pursuing my graduate work at the Palmer School of Chiropractic, the founding school of chiropractic medicine. Palmer is the highest ranked school in the field – and it is where my chiropractor had gone, and I wanted to be just like him if not better.

Upon graduation I received the award for Clinical Excellence throughout our entire clinic system, an award limited to five students. Today, I have multiple certifications in the wellness industry such as Functional Movement Specialist (FMS) and recently I have been accredited by the Better Business Bureau.

Do you think there is a difference for how women are treated when they are seeking help for ailments, and is it there a difference for women working in the wellness industry that brings some advantage/disadvantage?

The field of chiropractic medicine is heavily male dominated. I was one of six females in a class of 70. One day, we were in the palpation lab practicing on each other, and I had partnered up with Mark, who asked 'Where is the talus located?' I responded 'Here', pointing to the junction between the lower leg and ankle on the front side of the body. Mark ignored me and asked our male classmates until someone responded with the same answer I had given. I was like 'Why wouldn't you just listen to me?!' That's when I knew, as a female practitioner, that the chiropractic field would pose challenges.

I noticed that male chiropractors often rely on muscling through an adjustment, while women will be more precise, using physics to ensure the correct adjustment is done. Today, I still find it funny when a large male patient has the look of surprise on their face after they get an adjustment from me. I am only five feet tall and petite, so I need my adjustments to be as effective as my male colleagues.

Who inspires you in the wellness industry?

My mom has been an inspiration. When I was little, my mom suffered from chronic fatigue, severe depression, food allergies and an autoimmune condition (later diagnosed as Raynaud's). She tried acupuncturists for the depression and chronic fatigue, which provided her with some relief, but she eventually met a chiropractor who was able to help her further. The chiropractic adjustments meant that everything was working better – her vascular, neurological, and lymph systems. If I had not had that exposure to her holistic healing journey at such a young age, I may not have become a healer myself.

Can you provide some tips for our readers on how they can integrate wellness activities into their daily lives?

Soft tissue work is one of the best things anyone can do every day from the comfort of their home. My patients are shown how to use a foam roller and a massage ball to help increase their flexibility and mobility. While there might not be a ton of scientific research regarding the benefits of foam roller, every person I have worked with has noticed an immediate decrease in their pain.

The best part is it only requires about ten minutes of your time a day, and it's why I put together a 'Myofascial release guide' so people could benefit from using the foam roller and massage ball. It's a step-by-step guide that goes from head to toe with additional resources for some of the most common conditions our bodies may encounter.

If you were to describe how you feel about what it means to you to be sharing your love of wellness in three words, what would they be?

Passionate, comprehensive, healer.

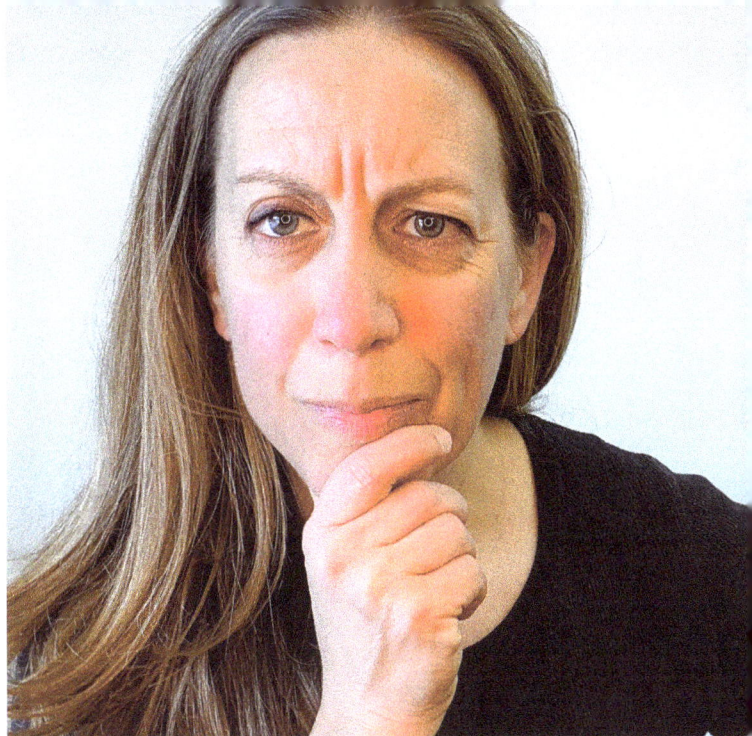

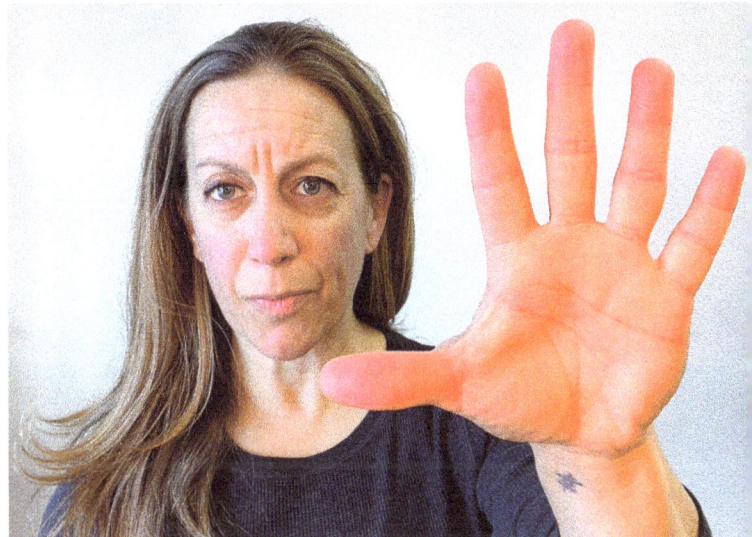

Is there anything else you would like to share with our readers?

If you are struggling with pain ... if you are wondering if you will ever be able to get back to the things you love most like running, playing golf or tennis, or playing with your children or grandchildren. If you are wondering if there is another option out there. Please accept my invitation to a free 30-minute video consultation with me. I am happy to help you put together the missing pieces, and provide you with an action plan to get you pain-free.

Explore ...

🌐 www.askdoctorheather.com

How did you get started in this area, what was the impetus to start doing what you do as a career choice? What sort of training/qualification did you need?

I have a Bachelor of Science in Human Biology and a Doctorate in Chiropractic Medicine. I am also trained in Biofeedback. Wellness has been a focus in my practice and has guided how I treat my patients. However, I don't think I truly realised the value of wellness until I became a patient myself. My illness caused me to lose my practice and put me in a situation where I was not able to work due to joint and muscle pain from rheumatoid arthritis and fibromyalgia. It was ultimately my own wellness practices that put me in a situation where I could go back to work.

Now I aid the elderly and disabled in finding the right advantage plan that will provide them with the best coverage. I focus on plans that approve wellness care and educate my clients on wellness uses.

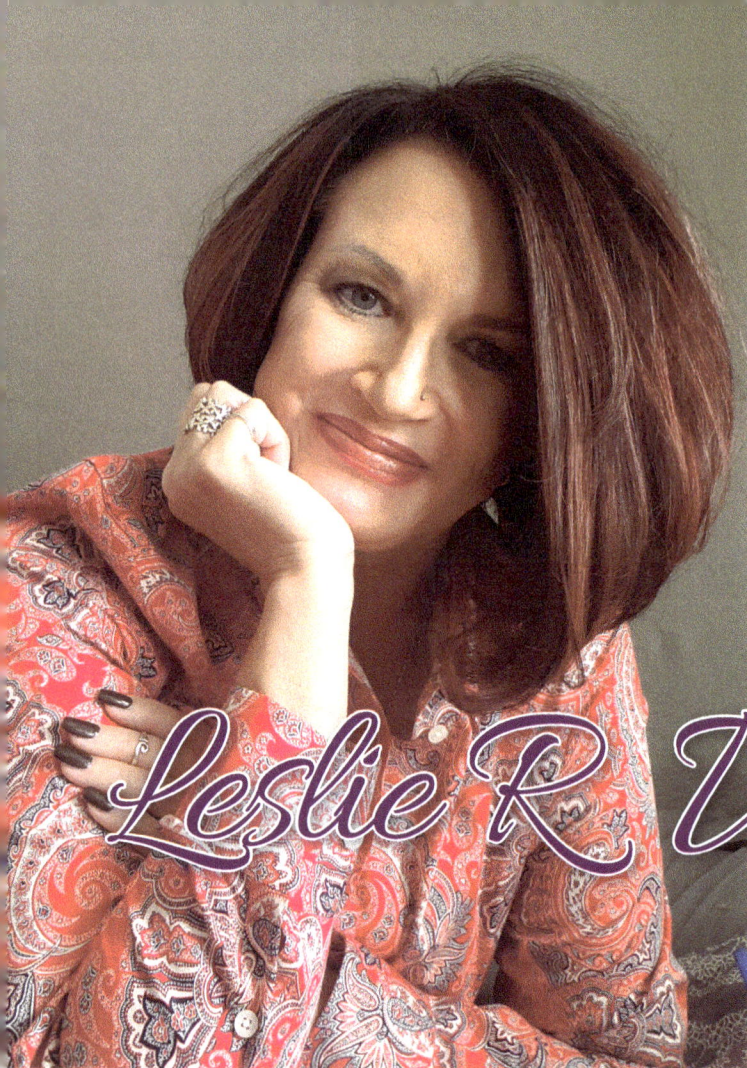

Leslie R Welch, DC

Author, Chiropractor, Mentor, Entrepreneur, Elder Insurance Producer, Welch Health Services

Tell us a bit about you, where you are located, and what is the work that you do as a woman working in the wellness industry?

Greetings! Well, I work in Oklahoma City, and I wear many hats. I am a chiropractor, an entrepreneur, a mentor, I do public speaking, and I am an insurance producer focusing on the elderly and the disabled.

Can you tell us a bit about your background? Has wellness always been an important focus for you?

I knew I wanted to be a doctor at 13, I just didn't know what kind of doctor. It was two ruptured discs, failed medical treatment, and successful chiropractic treatment that put me on the path of a wellness approach to medicine and to life.

Can you remember when you first realised that the wellness activity that you practice was an important part of your life? Was there an 'Aha!' moment like you'd solved a life puzzle?

I thought wellness was already part of my life – after all I dedicated my career to it as a chiropractor, but when I got rheumatoid arthritis (RA) and fibromyalgia, wellness in its many forms gave me my life back. It opened my eyes to its true power.

Do you think there is a difference for how women are treated when they are seeking help for ailments, and is it there a difference for women working in the wellness industry that brings some advantage/disadvantage?

Yes, I do! I experienced it myself as a patient. While being treated in Oklahoma City, I was treated with respect as I was already a respected part of the medical community, but when I sought a second opinion elsewhere, it was a whole different story. I could tell that the doctors didn't believe me before they even walked in the door. No one listened to anything I said. I felt like they thought of me as a complaining woman. It emotionally set me back, which is major when you have a disease and must deal with depression as well.

Who inspires you in the wellness industry?

Yes, definitely! Summer McStravick is the inventor of Flowdreaming and owner of Flowdreaming.com. She developed a manifesting technique that is easily incorporated into your day and very effective. She had cancer and was able to heal herself and took thousands of people along the journey with her. Her amazing intellect, her outstanding devotion to her members, and her con-tinued expansion of her program are inspiring. Her program changed my life, and after eight years I still use it on a regular basis.

Can you provide some tips for our readers on how they can integrate wellness activities into their daily lives?

I start with five minutes of meditation at the end of my bed every morning. You don't have to have a lot of money – you can do so many things by yourself. It just takes some

> I thought wellness was already part of my life – after all I dedicated my career to it as a chiropractor, but when I got rheumatoid arthritis (RA) and fibromyalgia, wellness in its many forms gave me my life back. It opened my eyes to its true power.

study and practice. Learn how to do Flowdreaming, study how to do biofeedback at home, read *Full Catastrophe Living* by John Kabat-Zinn, and incorporate mindfulness meditation into your life. Learn how to be in the moment. For example, when you are in the shower focus on being present. Feel the water, smell the soap, feel your wet hair and skin, recognise how you dry yourself off and see your routine intimately for the first time. Now apply that to your ailment. See it for the first time, recognise its patterns and realise that it is not you. Continue to search and try things, you never know what will help you.

If you were to describe how you feel about what it means to you to be sharing your love of wellness in three words, what would they be?

All that is!

Is there anything else you would like to share with our readers?

If I can help one person, it is worth it!

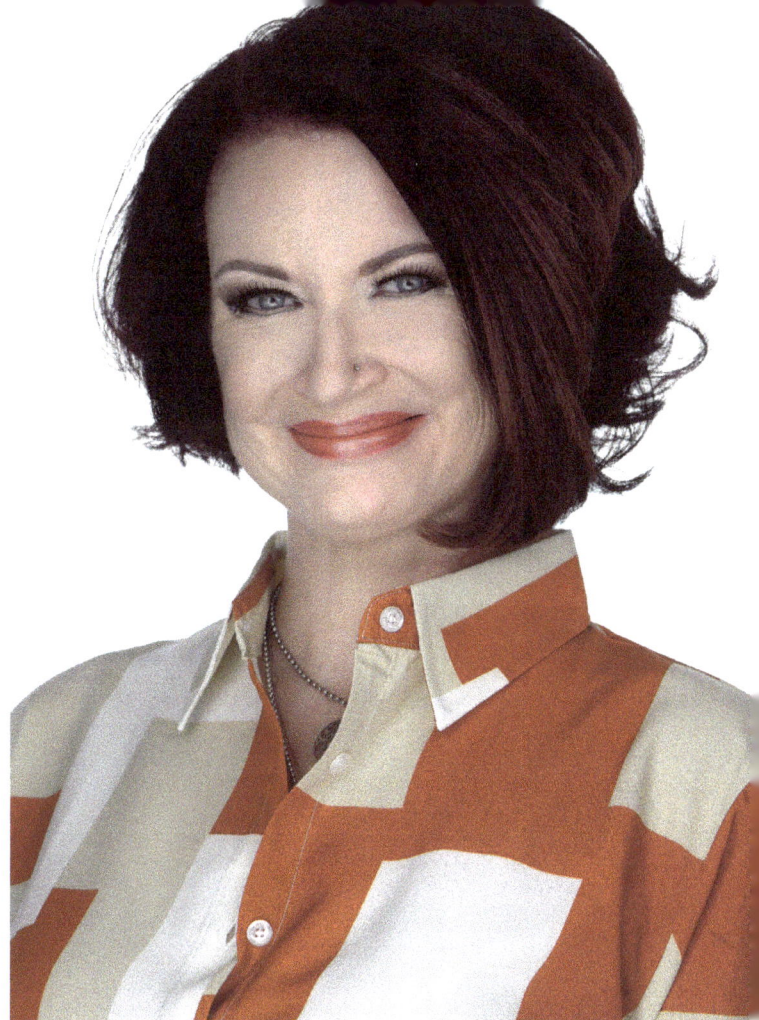

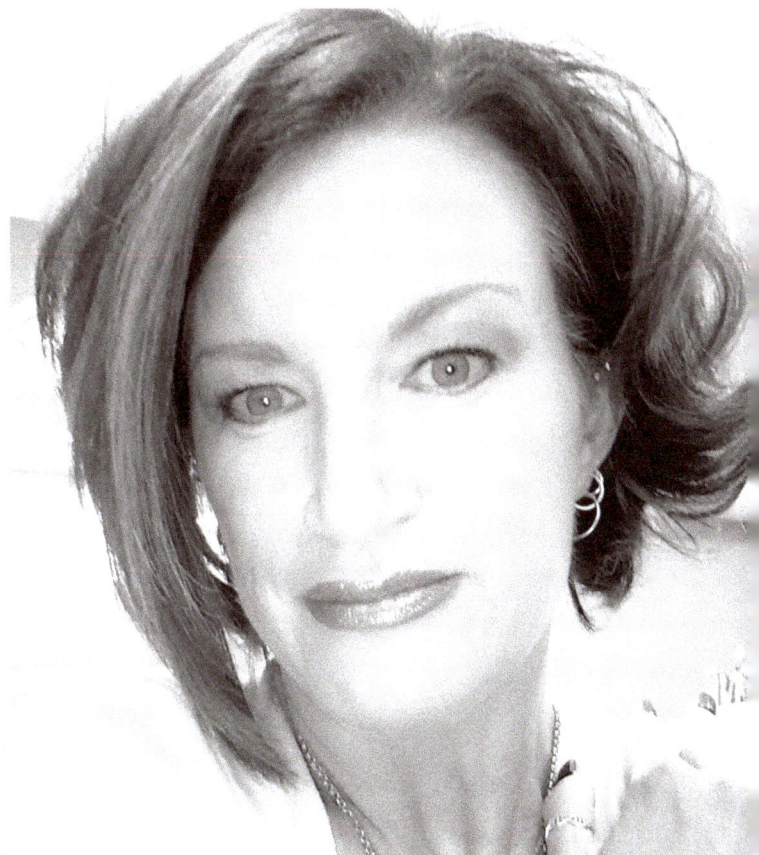

Explore ...

[instagram icon] www.instagram.com/leslierwelchdc

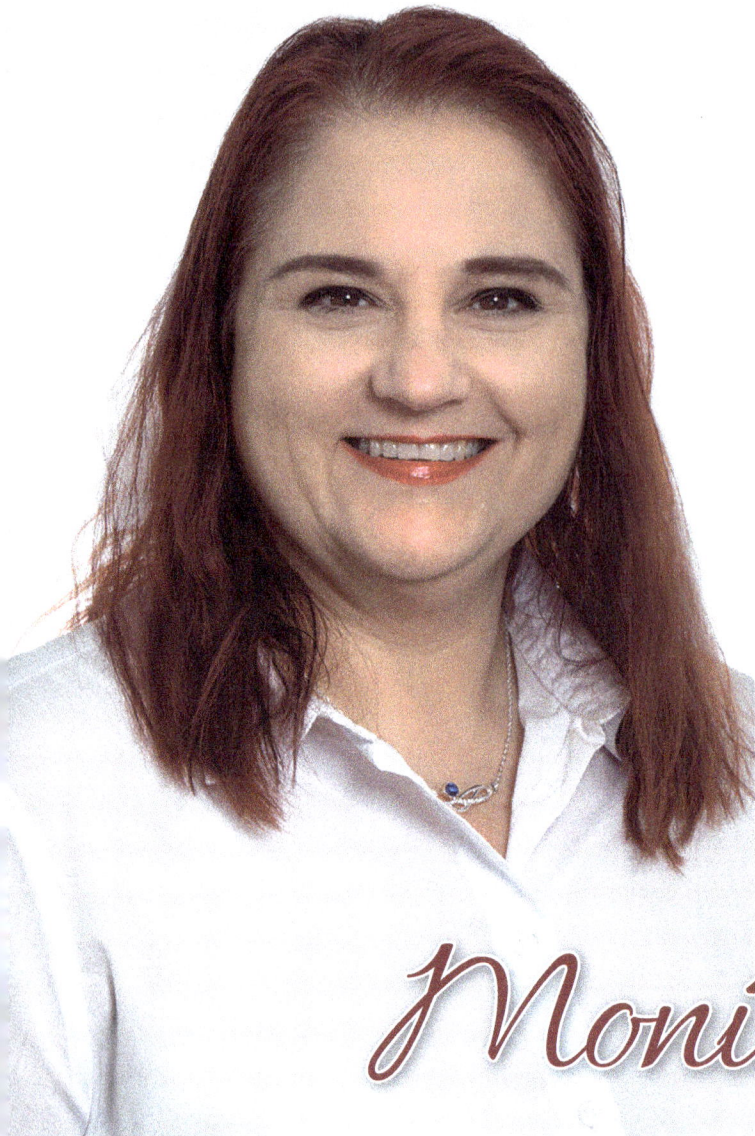

Can you tell us a bit about your background? Has wellness always been an important focus for you?

I am a trained conference interpreter and had been very analytical and rational before I fell ill. In 2009, I experienced some optical nerve issues and was diagnosed with multiple sclerosis (MS).

Today, I am grateful for my disease and diagnosis, as they launched me on the path of energy healing. With the threat of a so-called chronic, incurable disease over my head, I started questioning my life and the way I had looked at it so far. I was very grateful for the conventional medical therapies I was provided with, yet I also became curious about other ways to treat pain and illness. I trained as an energy healer and have continued to learn and evolve my spiritual and healing techniques. In 2017, I founded my small coaching and energy healing business. In 2020, I created my own healing modality, combining everything I had learned about the body and how to support our own healing powers.

Can you remember when you first realised that the wellness activity that you practice was an important part of your life? Was there an 'Aha!' moment like you'd solved a life puzzle?

When I started, I was looking for ways to help me manage my own MS journey. I was not envisioning having my own healing business. But then, my father underwent a difficult surgery, leaving him with a huge, painful scar. That was

Monika Korba

Self-Healing Mentor and Empowerment Coach.
Rise Up Coaching
Monika Korba

Tell us a bit about you, where you are located, and what is the work that you do as a woman working in the wellness industry?

I am a mom of two teenagers, and we live in beautiful Switzerland, close to Zurich, with its beautiful lakes and mountains.

As a woman working in the wellness industry, I support clients, mostly women, overcome their health issues such as chronic pain or chronic disease. Once we identify the root cause of the disease in their body, I help them transform it, so the body can activate its self-healing powers.

Our body is a miracle, and it can heal itself very well. Think about something as simple as a scratch or a cut, or a broken bone. The body can usually heal these very easily. On the other hand, healing yourself from a chronic ailment or pain can seem very difficult. We know the body can heal, but first we need to heal the hidden and trapped emotions that are keeping it stuck.

when I first tried energy healing on somebody else. And to my amazement, it worked! That was the moment I realised I had a gift, and I felt it would be selfish to not share this with the world.

How did you get started in this area, what was the impetus to start doing what you do as a career choice? What sort of training/qualification did you need?

What launched me on the path of energy healing, spiritual development, and ultimately women's empowerment, was my own experience with a so-called chronic disease. I have not had another attack or flare-up since my first in

2009. I was convinced I was able to help women in similar situations, not only regarding their health issues, but also teaching them how to truly reclaim their power in all areas of their lives. I had experienced how overwhelming life can become when you juggle family, work, friends, plus your own health issues. I had worked very hard on accepting and loving myself, stepping out of my victim mindset. I wanted to give other women the tools to do the same and create the life they want and deserve.

> I was convinced I was able to help women in similar situations, not only regarding their health issues, but also teaching them how to truly reclaim their power in all areas of their lives.

Do you think there is a difference for how women are treated when they are seeking help for ailments, and is it there a difference for women working in the wellness industry that brings some advantage/disadvantage?

Women are often not taken seriously when they talk about their health issues, especially when they talk about how they are feeling. Conventional medicine usually only looks at the physical aspects of an ailment. They will target the symptoms instead of looking at any wellbeing issue from a more holistic standpoint. The human being does not only consist of muscles, bones, and cells. We are so much more complex beings, and it is important to take all aspects of a person into account if we truly want to help them heal. Luckily, many people – men and women – are now taking a holistic approach, combining, for example, trauma-informed therapies with conventional medical techniques. It is true that this holistic approach is more often seen in women of the wellness industry, even though there are more men becoming aware that there is more than just the physical body. I definitely see progress here.

Who inspires you in the wellness industry?

The person who inspired me most was my general practitioner at the time of my diagnosis. He had a very down-to-earth approach, and he was combining different medical approaches, because he sent me to my first traditional Chinese medicine (TCM) therapy. There are many inspiring personalities in the wellness industry. You simply need to find those you resonate with most.

Can you provide some tips for our readers on how they can integrate wellness activities into their daily lives?

One of my favorite activities is gratitude, because it has the power to shift your mind from focusing on the negative to a more positive mindset. A positive mindset has a huge impact on our wellbeing. A positive mindset will reduce your stress level, helping reduce blood pressure and having a positive effect on your heart.

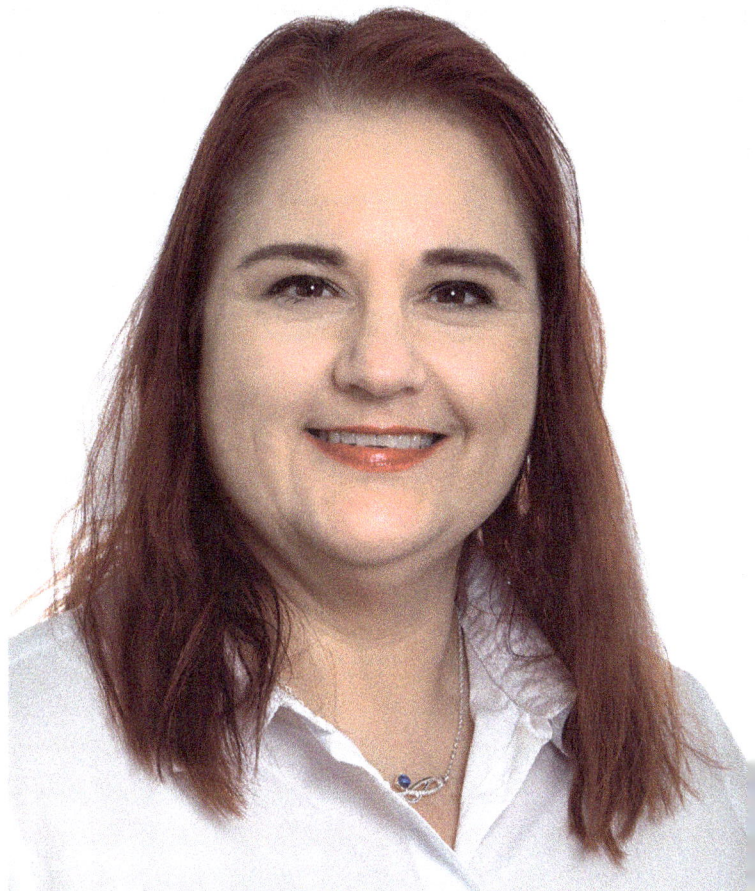

The next thing I use and love are breathing exercises. If you feel like you don't have the time, just take four deep breaths, counting to four when you inhale, holding your breath for four seconds, then slowly exhaling for four seconds. Deep breathing helps regulate the nervous system, reduces anxiety and stress, and can improve your mood. If you can combine it with light movements, like yoga or walking, even better. If you can't, just set your alarm during your lunch break to remind you to take a couple of deep breaths, and observe the effect this exercise will have on you.

If you were to describe how you feel about what it means to you to be sharing your love of wellness in three words, what would they be?

See others thrive.

Explore ...

🌐 www.rise-up-coaching.com

f www.facebook.com/riseupcoach.monika

📷 www.instagram.com/riseupcoaching_monika

Can you remember when you first realised that the wellness activity that you practice was an important part of your life? Was there an 'Aha!' moment like you'd solved a life puzzle?

Yes, I remember the moment when I realised that the wellness activities I was practicing were an important part of my life. I was struggling with anxiety and depression, and I was feeling hopeless. I started practicing meditation and visualisation, and I noticed a significant improvement in my mood and my overall wellbeing. I was feeling calmer, more focused, and more in control of my thoughts. I also realised that I was able to release stuck emotions that were contributing to my anxiety.

How did you get started in this area, what was the impetus to start doing what you do as a career choice? What sort of training/qualification did you need?

I got started in the wellness industry after my own experience with depression and anxiety. One day, I was introduced to the power of mindset and how our thoughts and beliefs can have a profound impact on our emotions

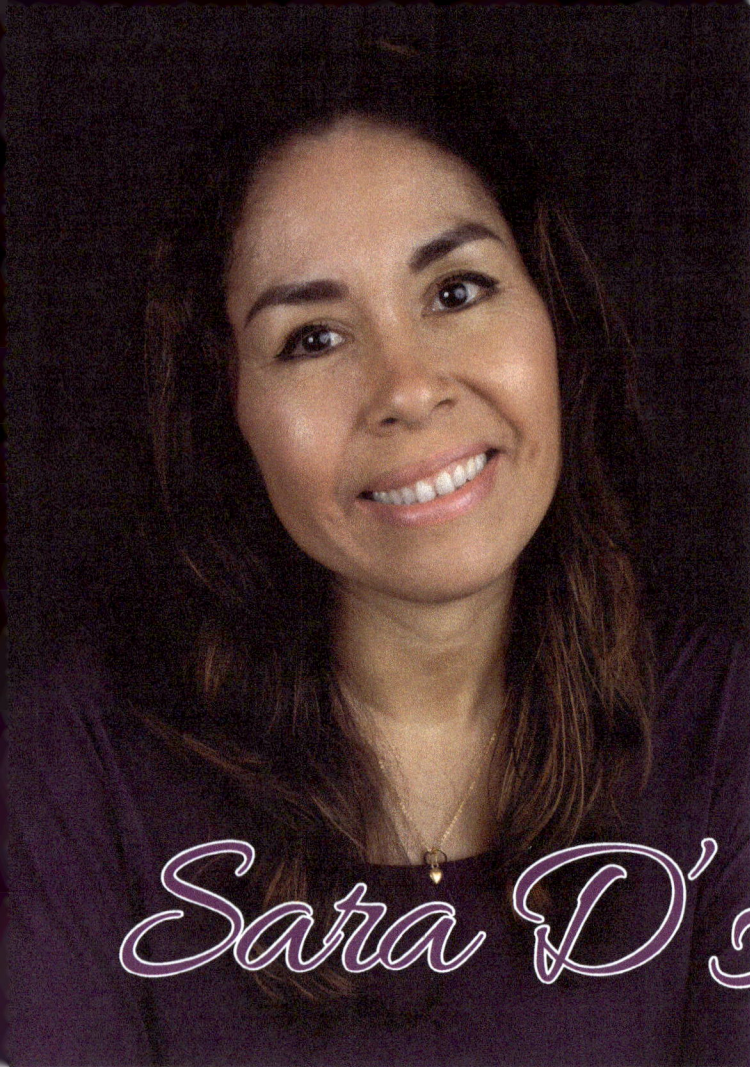

Sara D'Ambrosio

Mindset Coach and Author, Mastermind Products LLC

Tell us a bit about you, where you are located, and what is the work that you do as a woman working in the wellness industry?

I am a spiritual-personal development coach and author from Peru, living in Houston, Texas. I am passionate about helping others connect with their inner wisdom and tap into their full potential. I believe that everyone has the potential to live a life that is full of joy, love, and abundance.

Can you tell us a bit about your background? Has wellness always been an important focus for you?

I was born and raised in Peru. I studied hospitality management and always loved interacting with people from different cultures and backgrounds. I wanted to do something that would allow me to help others.

About 20 years ago, I got very sick and suffered from depression and anxiety. This was a challenging time for me, but it taught me a lot about myself and the power of the mind. I learned that I could control my thoughts and emotions, even when I was feeling physically unwell. I also learned the importance of taking care of my physical and mental health. After I recovered, I was determined to help others who were struggling with similar challenges.

and behaviours. As I started to change my thoughts and beliefs, I began to experience a dramatic improvement in my mental health.

I decided to become a life coach so that I could share my knowledge and experience with others. I am a certified coach, and I am always looking for new ways to improve my skills as a mindset coach.

Do you think there is a difference for how women are treated when they are seeking help for ailments, and is it there a difference for women working in the wellness industry that brings some advantage/disadvantage?

Yes, I believe that there is a difference for how women are treated when they are seeking help for ailments. Women's symptoms are often different from men's, which can lead to misdiagnosis or dismissal. For example, women are more likely than men to be told that their symptoms are 'all in their head' or that they are 'just being a hypochondriac'. This is a serious problem, as it can lead to women delaying or not seeking treatment for serious medical conditions.

Additionally, women working in the wellness industry may face advantages and disadvantages. On the one hand, women may be more likely to be seen as experts in wellness and connect with clients on a more personal level. However, they may also face challenges such as being paid less than men or being excluded from leadership positions.

Who inspires you in the wellness industry?

I am inspired by many people in the wellness industry, but two of my favorites are Bob Proctor and Kathleen Cameron. Bob is a self-help author and speaker who taught millions of people around the world how to achieve their goals. Kathleen was a nurse who became one of Bob's best students. She is an example of what it means to lead by example, and she has helped thousands of people transform their lives.

I admire their commitment to helping others. They have a genuine desire to see people succeed, and I am inspired by their example. I believe that everyone has the potential to achieve great things, and I am grateful to have learned from two of the most inspiring people in the wellness industry.

Can you provide some tips for our readers on how they can integrate wellness activities into their daily lives?

Here are some examples of wellness activities you can do.

Exercise: go for a walk, bike ride, or swim. Take a dance class or do yoga.

Healthy eating: eat plenty of fruits, vegetables, and whole grains. Limit processed foods, sugary drinks, and unhealthy fats.

Sleep: go to bed and wake up at the same time each day. Create a relaxing bedtime routine.

Relaxation: take a few minutes each day to relax and de-stress. Try meditation, yoga, or reading a book.

Social connection: spend time with friends and family. Get involved in your community.

The most important is to start small and gradually increase your activity level, find activities that you enjoy and make them a regular part of your routine, make it fun, and be patient with yourself.

If you were to describe how you feel about what it means to you to be sharing your love of wellness in three words, what would they be?

Passion, longevity, love.

Is there anything else you would like to share with our readers?

I would like to thank you for this opportunity to share my thoughts on wellness with you. I hope that you found this interview informative and inspiring. I encourage you to explore the many wellness activities that are available to you. You may be surprised at how much better you feel when you take care of yourself, physically and mentally.

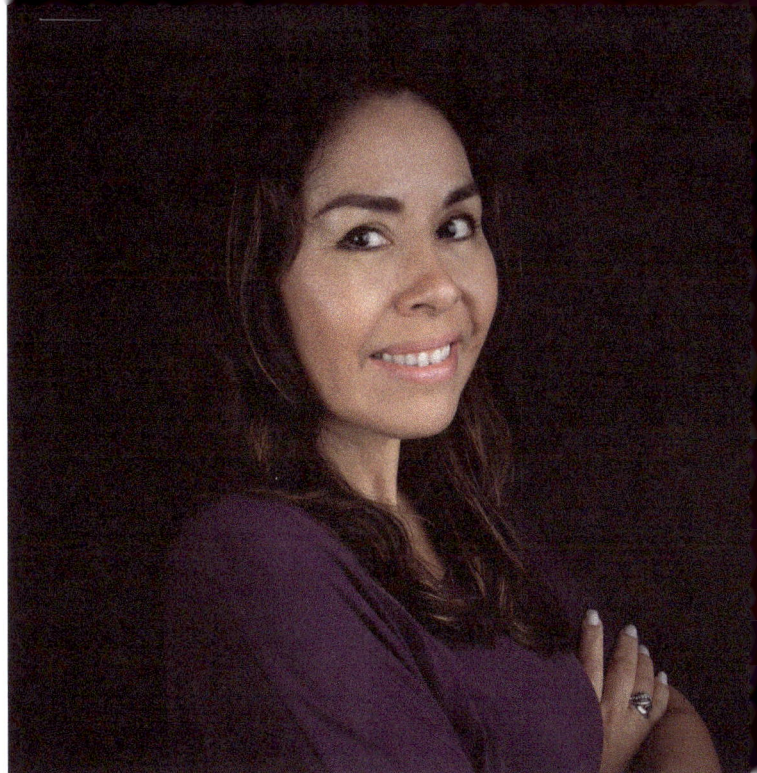

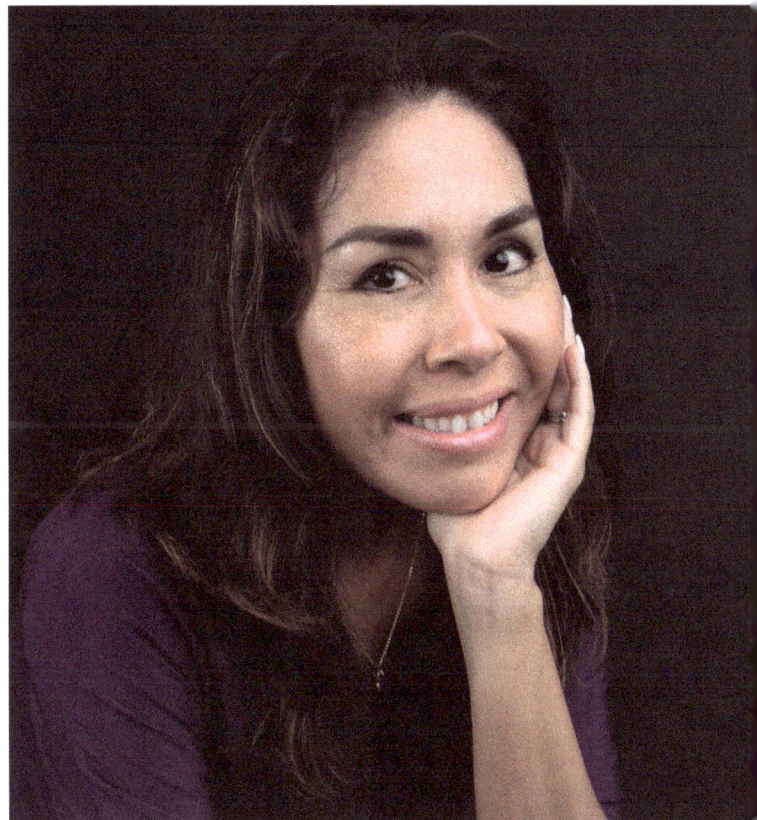

Explore ...

www.saradambrosiomastermind.com

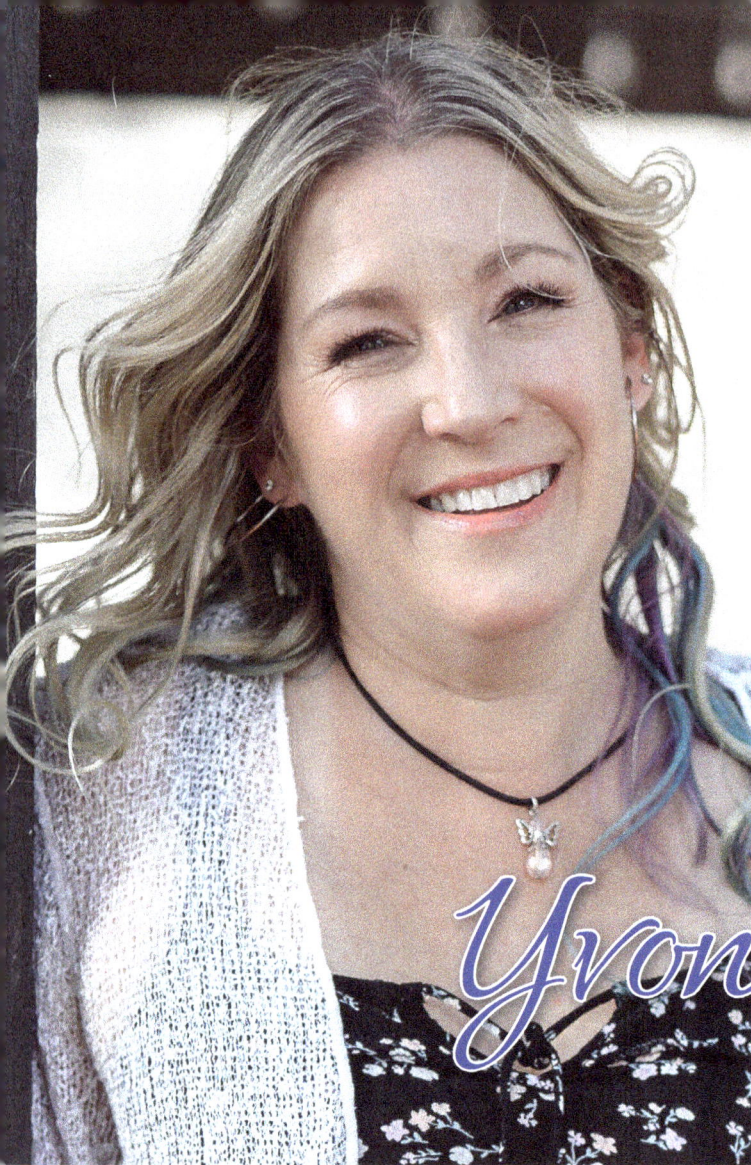

Yvonne Cote

Angel Medium and Spiritual Mentor, There is an Angel for That

Can you tell us a bit about your background? Has wellness always been an important focus for you?

As far back as I can remember, wellness has always played a big part in my life – personally and professionally. During my Human Resources career, a huge part of what I did entailed working with Health and Safety and Wellness. I always carried a belief in emotional, physical, and mental wellbeing. I had heard it said many times before that your place of business is only as good as its employees. Being in the role of Human Resources provided me with opportunities to consistently support individuals, including myself, in those areas. However, it wasn't until after my NDE, that I realised how important spiritual wellbeing is as well.

Can you remember when you first realised that the wellness activity that you practice was an important part of your life? Was there an 'Aha!' moment like you'd solved a life puzzle?

I was struggling with severe panic and anxiety, to the point of not wanting to leave my house. The medical system tried everything they could, but nothing was working for me. This went on for so long that I began to feel a sense of

Tell us a bit about you, where you are located, and what is the work that you do as a woman working in the wellness industry?

I am an Angel Medium and Spiritual Mentor based in Kelowna, BC, Canada. Following a near-death experience (NDE), I felt called to work with angels and have studied under renowned spiritual mentors to hone my talents. I hold multiple certifications as an Angel Practitioner and Guide, a Moonologist, Numerologist, and Colour Intuitive. I'm also a Reiki Master and a Crystal Healer.

Today, I share my passion for angels and their powers of healing, protecting, and guiding through private consultation where I specialise in helping people seeking clarity and alignment with their life purpose. I also host the 'There is an Angel for That' Podcast, where my esteemed guests and I offer tips on clearing energy and discuss how to utilise chakras to bring more balance to your life and connect with your angels. No matter what your situation, there IS an angel for it, and I can help you harness their power and guidance.

depression. I had lost a huge part of who I was as a person. I had normally been surrounded by people and places ... and this was now reduced to nothing.

My 'Aha!' moment came when I recalled a conversation I had with my emergency room doctor, following my NDE. He had made a comment that I was lucky to have survived, and that I must have had an amazing team of angels surrounding and supporting me. If those amazing angels did help save me that day like my doctor suggested, then was it possible that those same angels could help me release this panic and anxiety? It was in that moment that I felt my first signs of hope, and it was the beginning of my spiritual journey to health and wellness.

How did you get started in this area, what was the impetus to start doing what you do as a career choice? What sort of training/qualification did you need?

It wasn't until I started to explore the realm of spiritual hygiene and energy healing through modalities such as Reiki, Angels, Emotion Focused Therapy (EFT), and Color Therapy, that I was truly able to regain a state of wellness once more. This, by far, has been the biggest transformational shift I had ever achieved. I no longer suffered from panic and anxiety, and I slowly started to emerge back out into the world once more.

I was also eventually able to find my voice and learned by sharing my story that it was resonating with so many others. Almost all these conversations ended with 'Do you have you own business? Do you offer healing sessions or courses?' All this time, I had only ever considered my own healing/transformational journey, but that quickly shifted into me wanting to help others, and here I am today, living my life's true purpose!

If those amazing angels did help save me that day like my doctor suggested, then was it possible that those same angels could help me release this panic and anxiety?

Who inspires you in the wellness industry?

I have had the pleasure of being mentored by so many amazing teachers and coaches in the wellness industry, and I am so grateful for each and every one of them. However, someone who really inspired me was the late Louise Hay. Something really moved and shifted inside of me when I read her books, especially *You Can Heal Your Life*.

My biggest realisation came from learning the importance of self-love and self-care. Her message is very similar to what you hear when flying on a plane – that in the event of an emergency, you need to put on your oxygen mask first before assisting others. In other words, you won't be able to help others if you don't help yourself first. She also speaks of the importance of Gratitude, which is a practice I ensure I do several times a day, every single day.

Can you provide some tips for our readers on how they can integrate wellness activities into their daily lives?

Integrate something you like and want to do. Tap into your intuition, what feels good and what feels right for you? As well, start small by integrating only one or two things, and get comfortable doing them. As time goes on, you can always add in more.

If you were to describe how you feel about what it means to you to be sharing your love of wellness in three words, what would they be?

Grateful, empowering and expansive.

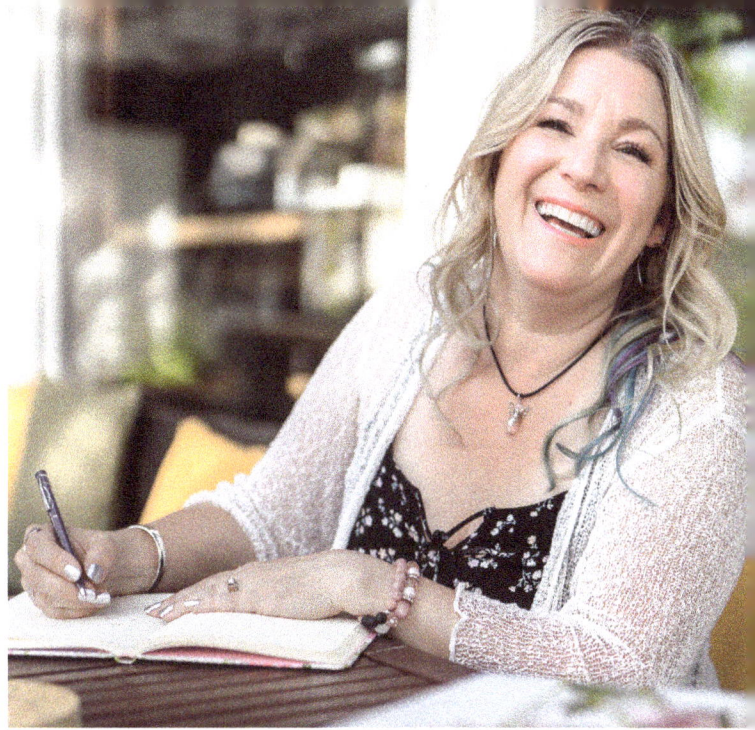

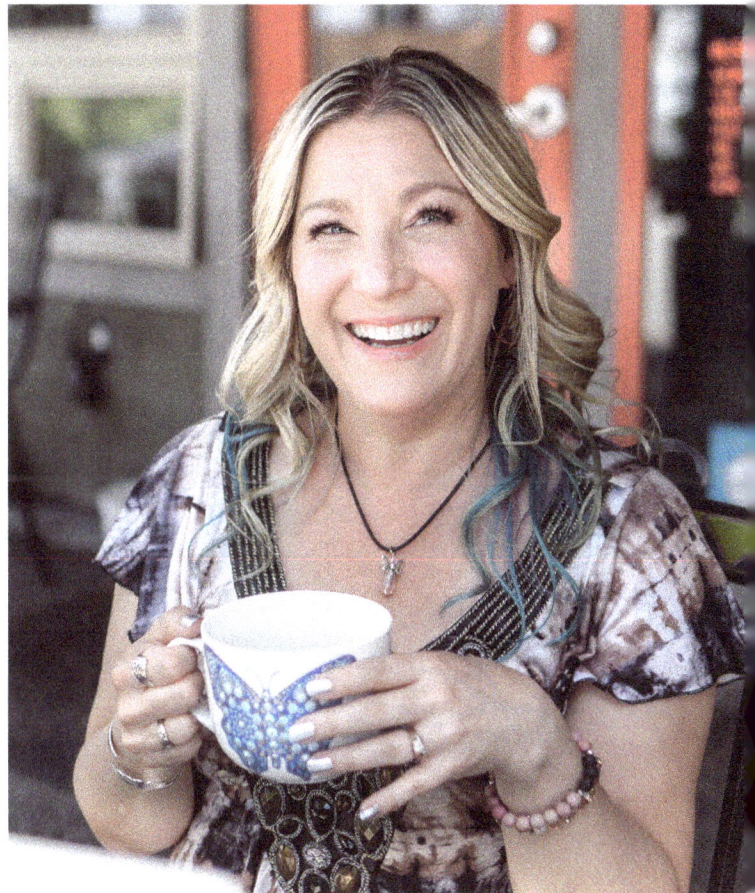

Explore …

🌐 www.thereisanangelforthat.com

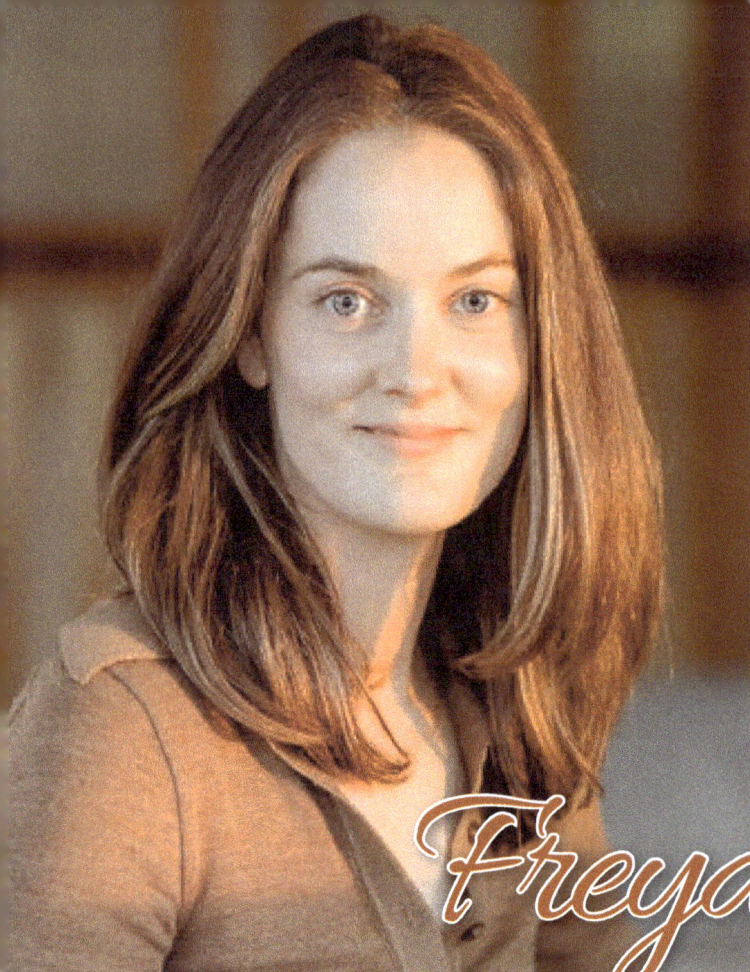

wellness was something that needed to be prioritised versus expected, and that medication wasn't always the only solution. I learned that, given the right environment, our bodies have the capacity to heal.

Can you remember when you first realised that the wellness activity that you practice was an important part of your life? Was there an 'Aha!' moment like you'd solved a life puzzle?

There are many. Moving from high intensity workouts to rejuvenating forms of exercise such as yoga and pilates. Cold plunging for a complete system reboot. Sauna and sweat-based therapies for detoxification and renewal. The list goes on. Whilst I don't prioritise one single modality, I know which one to lean on when my body needs it most.

How did you get started in this area, what was the impetus to start doing what you do as a career choice? What sort of training/qualification did you need?

Through my early exposure to naturopaths, homeopaths and natural healers, combined with my passion for sport and nutrition, studying to become a naturopath was the

Freya Lawler

Resident Naturopath and Nutritionist at Peninsula Hot Springs, Melbourne Freya Lawler Naturopathy

Tell us a bit about you, where you are located, and what is the work that you do as a woman working in the wellness industry?

I'm so excited to share my colourful journey with you. I am in beautiful Melbourne on the Yarra River, with nature and the city at my fingertips. I am a naturopath and nutritionist and primarily run my online virtual reproductive health clinic, which I love. I do get to enjoy the best of both worlds with virtual practice and face-to-face practice at Elgin House in Melbourne working alongside some of the best specialist gynecologists around. I also am a consultant for the Peninsula Hot Springs, and work as their resident naturopath and nutritionist. Throughout my entire degree, we were essentially told you will never make a great income or a good living from becoming a naturopath, and it became my mission to make sure this was not the case! There was also no conversation about other career opportunities outside of practicing one-to-one. I feel so fortunate to have experienced many different facets of being a naturopath. I have the best job in the world!

Can you tell us a bit about your background? Has wellness always been an important focus for you?

Growing up in stunning southern Tasmania, I was blessed to have been raised in a way that preferences holistic health versus conventional health as a number one priority. Through this early exposure, I learned that health and

most logical option. My family does not have an academic background, therefore a four-year Bachelor Degree felt unbelievably daunting to me. It took three visits to my university over a few years before I finally committed, but what a life changing decision it was. I feel unbelievably grateful to absolutely adore my career. It is really an extension of my life, which is the reality when you run your own business. However, I wouldn't have it any other way!

Do you think there is a difference for how women are treated when they are seeking help for ailments, and is it there a difference for women working in the wellness industry that brings some advantage/disadvantage?

I work specifically with reproductive health and endometriosis/chronic pelvic pain, so there is absolutely a disparity in healthcare for men and women. Women are more likely to be disbelieved and denied treatment than men, even though women are far more likely to be suffering from chronic pain. There is also a disparity in high quality research. Most of the research is conducted on men, which in many circumstances is not transferable to the female population.

The stories of medical gaslighting are countless, especially when it comes to chronic pain. Much of my work includes coaching patients on how to be their own health advocate. It's unfortunate, but necessary, especially when you aren't getting answers to your chronic health concerns.

Who inspires you in the wellness industry?

Any woman or individual assigned female at birth (AFAB) who is working to break the taboos around reproductive health care. Chronic pelvic pain is not normal. Huge shifts in mood before your period are not normal! Women and AFAB individuals are in pain during their periods, or all throughout the month, while having sex they experience pain, coupled with hormonal migraines, premenstrual syndrome (PMS)/premenstrual dysphoric disorder (PMDD), headaches, joint aches, painful bladders, irritable bowels, sore lower backs, muscle pain, vulval pain, vaginal pain, jaw pain, and muscle aches. And many are unbelievably tired. Sadly, this pain is all too often dismissed, and their illnesses misdiagnosed or ignored. So, thank you to all of the incredible humans out there breaking the taboos and giving women and those AFAB the confidence to stand up for themselves and seek the care they truly need.

Can you provide some tips for our readers on how they can integrate wellness activities into their daily lives?

1. Tune into your body. Take note of the signs and symptoms you are experiencing. This is your body's way of communicating with you. Ideally, we avoid band aiding these signs and symptoms, but rather enquire as to what might be causing this dysfunction. And please don't settle for 'It's normal'. Listening to your body is an amazing act of self-care and one that can bring such profound benefits. Our body doesn't lie.

2. Get curious. Experiment with various wellness activities and see which one you love or the one that makes you feel the best. Stick with that.

3. Start switching your drinks with the girls to a bathing session at the Hot Springs or a bathhouse like Sense of Self in Collingwood – a place where you can deeply connect whilst experiencing the restorative and rejuvenating aspects of geothermal bathing and sauna. And you feel fantastic the next day!

If you were to describe how you feel about what it means to you to be sharing your love of wellness in three words, what would they be?

Joyous, enriching, honoured.

Is there anything else you would like to share with our readers?

Thank you so much for sharing this really important information with your wider audience!

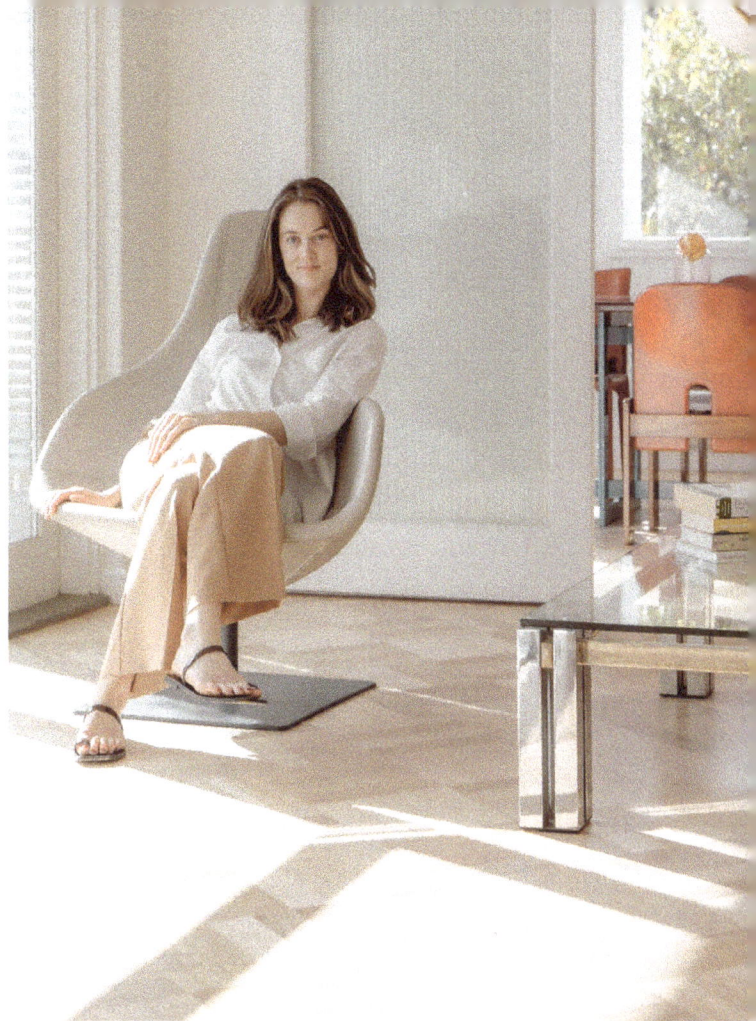

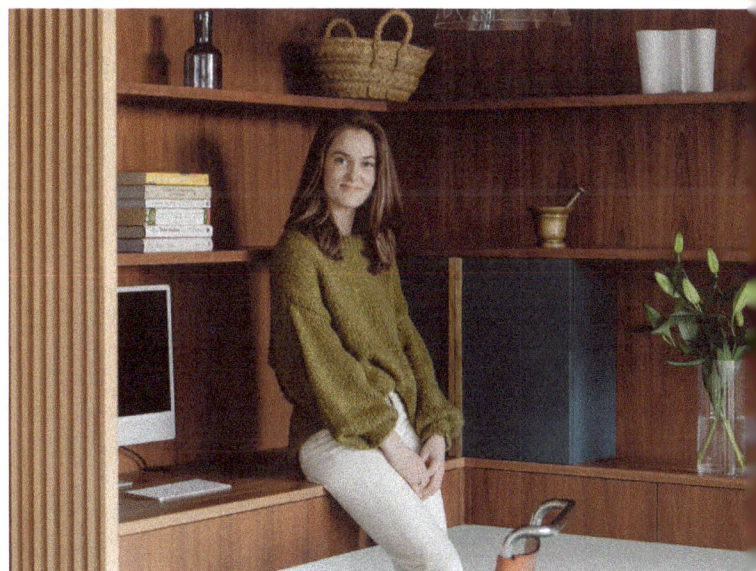

Explore ...

www.instagram.com/freyalawlernaturo

www.freyalawler.com.au

Kerry Thurrowgood

LōKAHI Wellness CEO

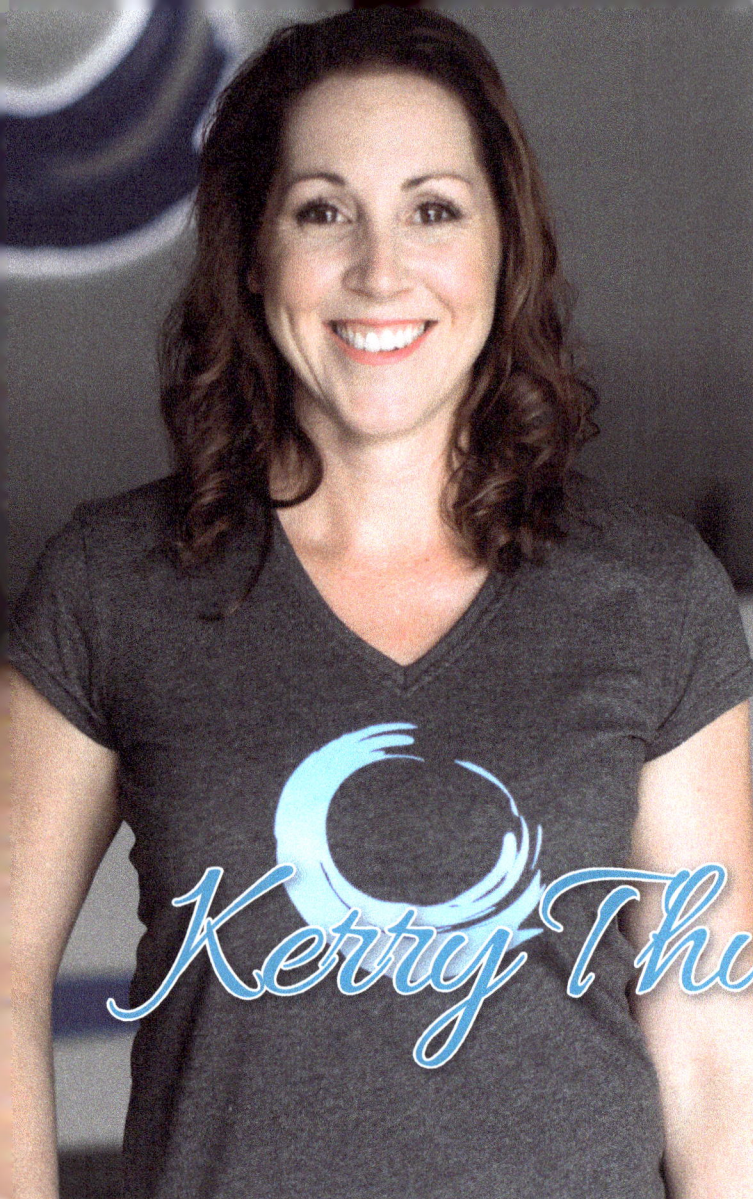

Can you tell us a bit about your background? Has wellness always been an important focus for you?

I am originally from the Bahamas and have lived in many different places. I have experienced lots of different cultures and different ways that people look after themselves, and this helps me in the work I do now. As a child, I was a swimmer and into lots of different sports at a competitive level and understood the importance of recovery and keeping my mind right to compete at my best.

I have been in the wellness industry for over 20 years, and prior to this I was a Personal Trainer and Health coach who specialised in autoimmune conditions, with a focus on Hashimoto's disease. We are more than just physical, and whilst eating right and training is important, there are also mental and spiritual aspects to our health. Because of this I studied many different modalities, including iridology, and I am also a Reiki master.

I love learning about our body and am in awe of what our bodies and minds can overcome given the opportunity. I am incredibly blessed as I feel I am living my life's purpose every day.

Tell us a bit about you, where you are located, and what is the work that you do as a woman working in the wellness industry?

My name is Kerry, and I have a beautiful family – my husband Scott and our five children. I am also co-founder and CEO of LōKAHI Wellness. LōKAHI Wellness is in Kilsyth South in the eastern suburbs of Melbourne, and we are one of the largest wellness centres in Australia.

Our pain management and stress relief treatments include float therapy, infrared saunas, cryotherapy, mild hyperbaric oxygen therapy (mHBOT), Normatec lymphatic sessions, cyclic variations in adaptive conditioning (CVAC), massage, and a range of practitioners.

I have always had an interest in health and wellness and helping people, but our concept for this business came because Scott had a back injury and everything we've included in the centre are things that helped him.

Our mission is that everyone that comes into our centre feels better.

Can you remember when you first realised that the wellness activity that you practice was an important part of your life? Was there an 'Aha!' moment like you'd solved a life puzzle?

My 'Aha!' moment was realising I AM worth giving myself time for wellness. For a long time, I didn't think I was worth putting time aside for my wellness. But for me to be able to help my family, my friends and our clients, I must put time aside for my wellness. I am no good to anyone if I am not well. I also want my children to model looking after themselves so they can be the best versions of themselves.

Give yourself permission to feel good.

How did you get started in this area, what was the impetus to start doing what you do as a career choice? What sort of training/qualification did you need?

Our catalyst was Scott's back injury. He went from being a roof tiler and body builder – incredibly independent, fit, and healthy – to not being able to work and needing assistance in getting dressed. Seeing how debilitating the chronic pain was for him physically and mentally was extremely tough. His neurologist told him that he should just take pain killers until he has surgery. Whilst medication has its place, being on pain killers permanently wasn't the answer for us, and we started looking for alternatives. We started with an infrared sauna. The infrared wavelengths helped reduce his pain, and he could dress himself after a session.

A friend told us to try a float tank. Float tanks are filled with 500kg of magnesium, which helps with muscle relaxation and recovery, nerve pain, anxiety and depression. When he floated, it was the first time he had been pain-free since his injury. For someone that lived with an 8 out of 10 pain every day, to have no pain was incredible.

Having actively started looking for alternative therapies, we found cryotherapy, and after his sessions his pain would decrease from 8/10 to 3/10.

In February 2017, we were about to make the hour's drive so he could have a float and Scott said, 'I wish this was closer'. I responded with 'How good would it be if everything was closer'. We looked at each other and said 'We should do that!' Exactly one year later we opened.

It's funny how things work. The tragedy that was his back injury became our greatest gift.

Do you think there is a difference for how women are treated when they are seeking help for ailments, and is it there a difference for women working in the wellness industry that brings some advantage/disadvantage?

The most common thing I hear from women is they do not feel heard. There seems to be a real issue with band-aid approaches or numbing of the problem, instead of getting to the root of the issue. They are told they are 'hormonal' or 'depressed', when in fact things are going on that should not be ignored. What's worse is these women are putting up with horrible symptoms until it gets so bad with so many issues snowballing, it becomes a serious health crisis.

My distinct advantage being a woman in the wellness industry is that people will share what is going on for them. I hear them and refer them on to specialists that I know will help. I don't know if the same level of honesty would happen with clients if I was a man.

Who inspires you in the wellness industry?

Nat Kringoudis is a Women's Health Practitioner who works incredibly hard to help women.

Can you provide some tips for our readers on how they can integrate wellness activities into their daily lives?

Start by breathing. Take seven deep breaths in and out. Allow five minutes for your wellness practice each day, and build from there. Find what works for you. Look for experiences you enjoy – walks in the bush, meditation, ice baths, infrared saunas.

Make sure you get more magnesium into your body. Try floating, I promise it will make a difference. Most importantly, give yourself permission – you are worth it.

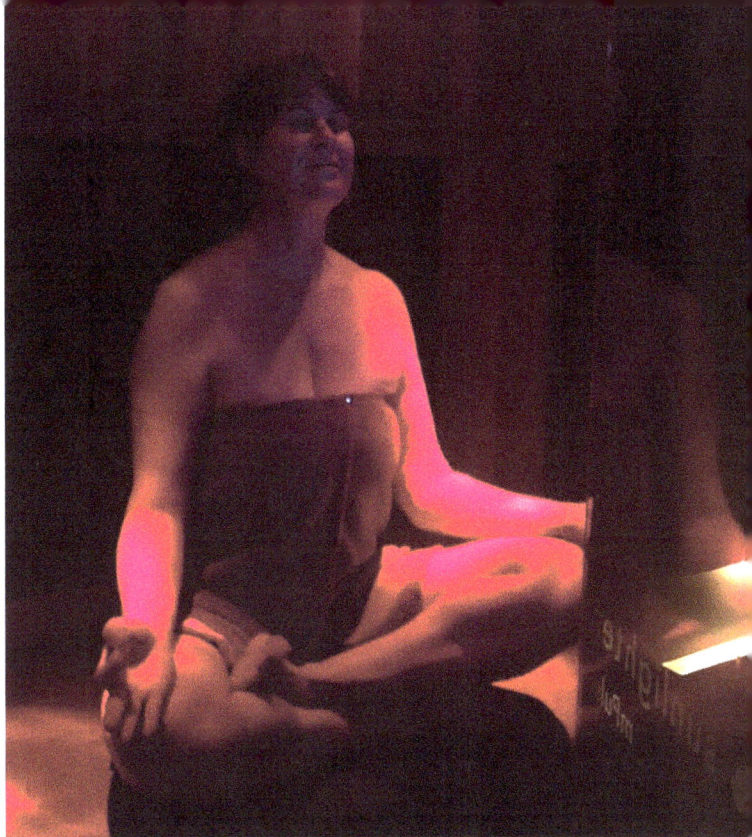

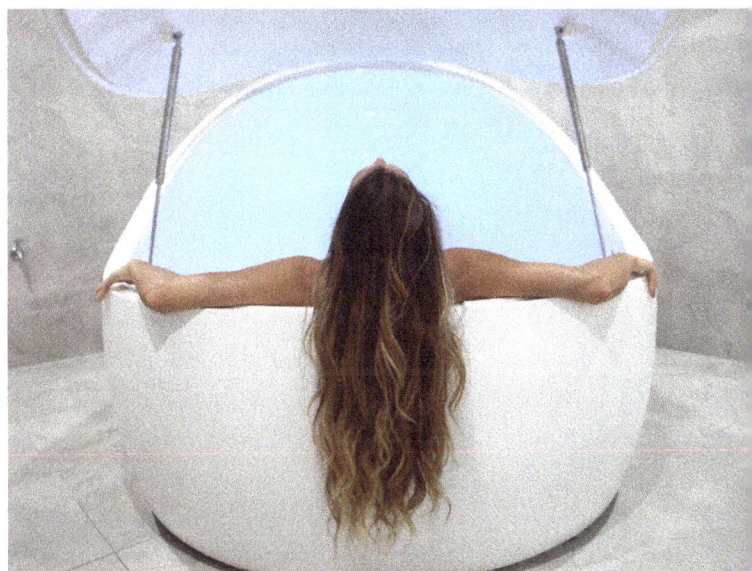

If you were to describe how you feel about what it means to you to be sharing your love of wellness in three words, what would they be?

Living my purpose.

Explore ...

🌐 www.lokahiwellness.com.au

Take time to
breathe

Breathing is an innate skill.

We took our first breath to enter this world.

We can go for days without food and water,
but only minutes without breath.

Many of us are not breathing properly.
Good breathing helps us to relax, regulates our system,
supplies oxygen to our cells and our brain. Check in with
yourself during the day. Many of us shallow breathe when we
are stressed, and often by the end of the day many of us are
shallow breathing.

Check yourself.

Are you only breathing down as far as your chest?

Take some time to be still and concentrate on your breathing.
Gentle slow breaths right down to your belly.

Scan our QR code to access our free
'Wellness on Time' belly breathing meditation

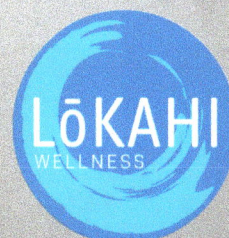

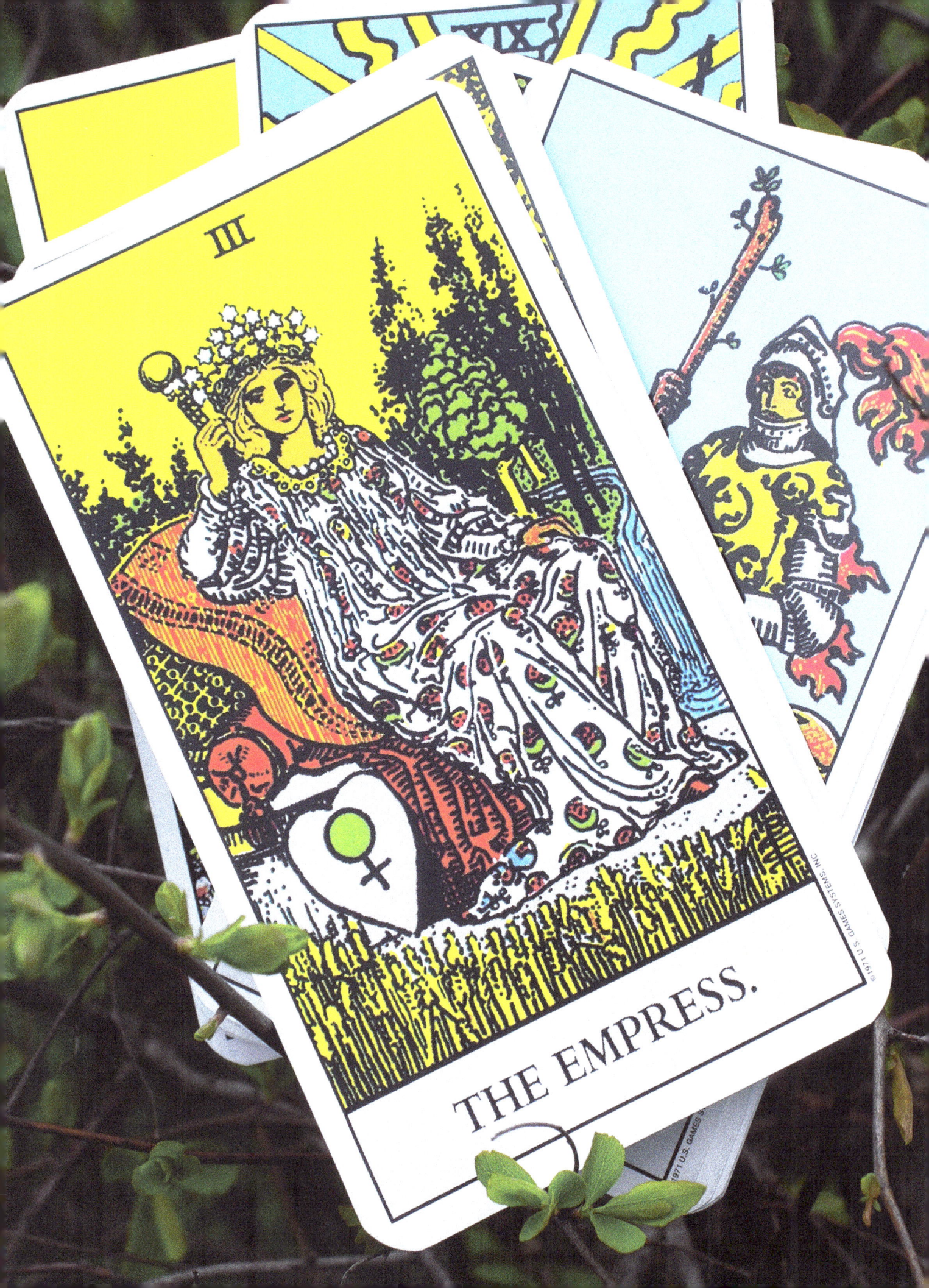

III

THE EMPRESS.

Beyond fortune telling: harnessing the power of tarot for personal growth

By Amanda Doyle

If you're in the spiritual space, you've heard of tarot reading. It's a practice that involves using a deck of tarot cards to gain insight and guidance. It's often used as a tool for exploring various aspects of a person's life, seeking answers to specific questions, and gaining a deeper understanding of the world or what might happen. You may not realise that you can use tarot to gain a deeper understanding of yourself.

Tarot can be used as a tool for self-discovery and personal growth – it is not solely about fortune telling but can be used as a powerful means of self-reflection and understanding. In this article, I will outline three ways that you can use tarot as a tool for self-discovery and reflection instead of just looking for answers to questions you may not need to know the answer to.

The first thing you can do is explore archetypal energies. Try to discover yourself through the deck. In each tarot deck, there are archetypal energies present. Each card has a specific message and energy that relates to it. In fact, a lot of the cards have people on them. Each tarot card can represent a different aspect of the human psyche.

One thing you can do is ask the deck for cards that resonate with your personal journey and reflect on how these energies manifest in your life. Let's say you pull 'The Empress'. This means that you are a nurturing person, and you care a lot about the people around you – but something you may have to watch out for is to make sure you're not smothering the people that you love. When you can recognise and integrate these energies into your life, you can find more balance.

A beneficial practice is incorporating tarot into your daily routine. You do this by drawing one card each morning, and then taking the time to observe the symbolism of the card, as well as the emotions and thoughts that come up for you when you see this card.

Reflect on how the card relates to your current life circumstances and observe the deeper meaning. I suggest keeping a notebook to put these reflections in, which can be kept as a memento to help you discover more about yourself over time.

An interesting way to incorporate tarot into your life is to use tarot as a guide for personal growth. Try selecting a card that represents a trait or quality that you admire or wish to develop. Let's say you want to be like 'The Empress' – you want to be that nurturing and loving person. When you take the energy of the card and engage in activities or practices that embody the essence of the chosen card, you can transform. If you want to embody the energy of 'The Empress', you could do things that are more nurturing to the people around you. If you want to embody the energy of 'The Emperor', you can start to become more of a leader in your life.

I want you to remember that tarot is personal. It is meant to be subjective. Connect to your intuition and find methods that resonate with your individual preferences. Tarot should be a unique experience that fills you with satisfaction, not anxiety.

I encourage you to experiment and explore different tarot spreads, rituals, or practices that enhance your self-discovery process. Try some of these activities and see how you can use tarot in a new way.

Tarot may seem scary, but if you use your intuition and trust your own interpretations and insights, you can use this as a tool for self-discovery, not just fortune telling.

Tarot cards have huge potential as a tool for reflection, as you can use them to discover the energies that reside within you that need to be balanced, uncover hidden parts of yourself, and guide you on a path to success.

Tarot cards can be transformative, and if you incorporate them into your wellness and self-improvement journey, you might be surprised.

Through regular engagement with the tarot deck, you can deepen your understanding of yourself, cultivate self-awareness, and embark on a path of personal growth and self-development.

So, what are you waiting for? The cards are calling your name!

Amanda is a life coach, tarot reader and founder of Happily Mander – explore self-discovery through tarot readings and tarot coaching.

Support your immune system with a balanced approach

Immunity in a COVID-19 world – it's the hot topic on many people's lips. How to improve it, what to eat to boost it, and what supplements will help strengthen it. All too often we're told it's our diet that makes the biggest amount of difference when it comes to our immunity, but there is a lot more to it than just getting your 'five-a-day'. A well-functioning immune system is born from a state of balance in mind, body and nutrition.

How does the immune system work?

'Virus and bacteria are still a part of our environment, it is just we have to learn how to relate to them so they don't affect us any more. This is what our bodies have been designed to do. Our body is forced to learn how to relate to everything foreign that it takes in. All systems in our body including gastrointestinal, circulatory, immune and lymphatic systems need to function well for this process to occur,' Chinese acupuncturist Brigitte Lalor explains. 'If the whole body is functioning efficiently, we have a strong immune system.'

Brigitte works in the field of Chinese medicine, which takes a holistic view of the body, 'Inspecting the exterior to examine the interior'. Unlike traditional medicine, it looks at the derivatives of pain and illness, seeking to find the underlying malfunction rather than just treat acute symptoms. The immune system plays a major role in this. For example, you might often get coughs, colds or bugs and always just use cold and flu tablets to keep them at bay.

The more important issue to look at here would be the immune system – why is it not functioning as it should, and what elements of your lifestyle might be damaging it? Fixing the immune system and surrounding lifestyle choices ensures a longer-term solution, potentially preventing not just one instance of a cold, but a multitude of other illnesses in the future.

This is where the 'holistic' view of your body and health comes in. Immunity can be affected by a whole range of factors – stress, smoking, alcohol consumption, sedentary lifestyles, over-exercising and even grief. To help your immune system, it's about being honest with yourself about what aspects of your lifestyle might need changing in order to restore balance in your body.

How can I make changes to benefit my immune system?

We're going to cover some things to think about when it comes to making changes. But of course, please speak to a doctor or health professional if you are having symptoms of any type of illness, or if you're thinking of making drastic changes.

1. Stress

This is one of the biggest and least talked about contributors to a weakened immune system. When we are stressed, our body produces the hormone corticosteroid. This hormone suppresses the effectiveness of the immune system, reducing its ability to fight off antigens. In times like this, where stress is heightened for many of us, it's really important to take time to actively relax. By that, we mean taking steps to reduce your screen time, spend time in nature and do whatever activities help you to slow down. It might be taking a walk, knitting, dancing, yoga or meditation. Although sweating it out might be one of your key ways of releasing stress, consider swapping one or two high-intensity interval training (HIIT) or endurance exercise sessions with a more gentle form of exercise. Also, share your stress with others. Whether it's with a loved one or over a video call with a friend, having an open dialogue about your stress levels is really important. However, seeking professional advice is also an important step.

2. Strengthen your weaknesses

'To have good health, look at where your body is struggling or not functioning well, and take action to improve those areas', says Brigitte. 'For example, symptoms of bloating after eating and food moving really slowly through the body may impact the production of new healthy cells. Symptoms of laboured breathing and shortness of breath will diminish energy levels, as cells need oxygen to convert glucose into energy. If we strengthen the body's weakness, we are supporting the body to function more efficiently and effectively.'

So, this means examining your body and its functions – if you do have symptoms, what do they point towards? Maybe you've put up with bloating but never really done anything to change it – gut issues could be a key part of why

your immune system isn't functioning optimally. Do your research. Speak to medical professionals and look to other types of healing such as Chinese medicine, daily Tai Chi/Qi Gong, breath-work, and meditation to find what works for you.

3. Mindful movement

As we mentioned before, movement plays a huge role in our overall stress levels and therefore our immunity. However, this extends out from just the forms of exercise we engage in on a daily basis. Being sedentary throughout the day, without much movement except from your allotted exercise time, can negate many of the benefits exercise gives us when it comes to our overall health. At the 'Evidence-based integrated healthcare' symposium hosted by RMIT University, Professor Neville Owen, Head of the Behavioural and Generational Change Program at the Baker IDI Heart and Diabetes Institute, told guests that, '... excessive sitting time – whether in front of a television or at the desk – was emerging as a new risk factor for chronic disease.' So what can you do? It's pretty simple. Make sure you take breaks from your work throughout the day. Setting a timer for hourly breaks is a great way to get into the habit of stretching your legs throughout your day.

4. The old favourite – nutrition

Finally, a quick dip into nutrition. Of course this does have a role to play, but it's not easily fixed by just gulping down some supplements or an immunity juice.

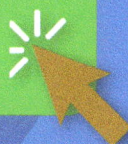

4 spices
to boost your immunity

Spices. For most in the western world, they're a sure-fire way to inject some flavour and depth into a dish. However, in many cuisines, the use of spices is intrinsically tied to their use in ancient medicine. Although 'modern medicine' has arguably overridden these ancient forms of medicine, there has been extensive research on the benefits of spices that still stand today. So, we've picked out the top four immune-boosting spices for you and some recipes to help you integrate them into your everyday.

Turmeric

The magic compound in turmeric is curcumin, a powerful antioxidant and anti-inflammatory. The antioxidants help to fight infection and the anti-inflammatory qualities help to relieve the body from cold and flu symptoms.

Be sure to pair it with black pepper, which is full of piperine – the key to helping your body absorb the effects of curcumin.

1. **Turmeric latte.** Heat your favourite milk and add ½ tsp turmeric powder, a grind of black pepper, and your sweetener of choice.

2. **Turmeric and pear porridge.** Heat your milk of choice milk and oats together in a saucepan. Add a ½ tsp turmeric and a grind of black pepper. Once getting thick, swirl through some honey and top with sliced pear.

3. **Turmeric and tahini dip.** Combine ½ cup tahini with 2 teaspoons of turmeric, black pepper, salt, 1 clove of grated garlic, a splash of vinegar and a little water. Serve with any salad, falafels, or as a dip with crudités.

Cinnamon

Cinnamon is packed with antioxidants that have fantastic effects on the immune system. It can reduce inflammation and potentially increase immune cell production, making it a must-include spice when you're feeling a little under the weather.

1. **Veggie stew.** Chop some of your favourite veggies (we love onions, carrots, zucchinis and pumpkin) and put them into a pot. Add water to cover and 2 tsp cinnamon, salt, pepper, 1 tsp dried cumin, 3 cloves of crushed garlic, 2 tsp dried oregano and bring to the boil. Once the vegetables are semi-soft, add some canned and washed beans or lentils. Stir to combine and serve with crushed nuts and seeds or bread.

2. **Blueberry pie smoothie.** Add 1 ½ cups of frozen blueberries, ice, ½ frozen banana, almond milk and ½ tsp cinnamon to a blender. Blend until smooth.

3. **Cinnamon sweet potatoes.** Cube up 2 large sweet potatoes, spread on a baking tray and drizzle with olive oil. Sprinkle over cinnamon and salt, mix to combine so all cubes are coated in the oil, cinnamon and salt. Bake in a medium heat oven for 30–45 minutes until crisp.

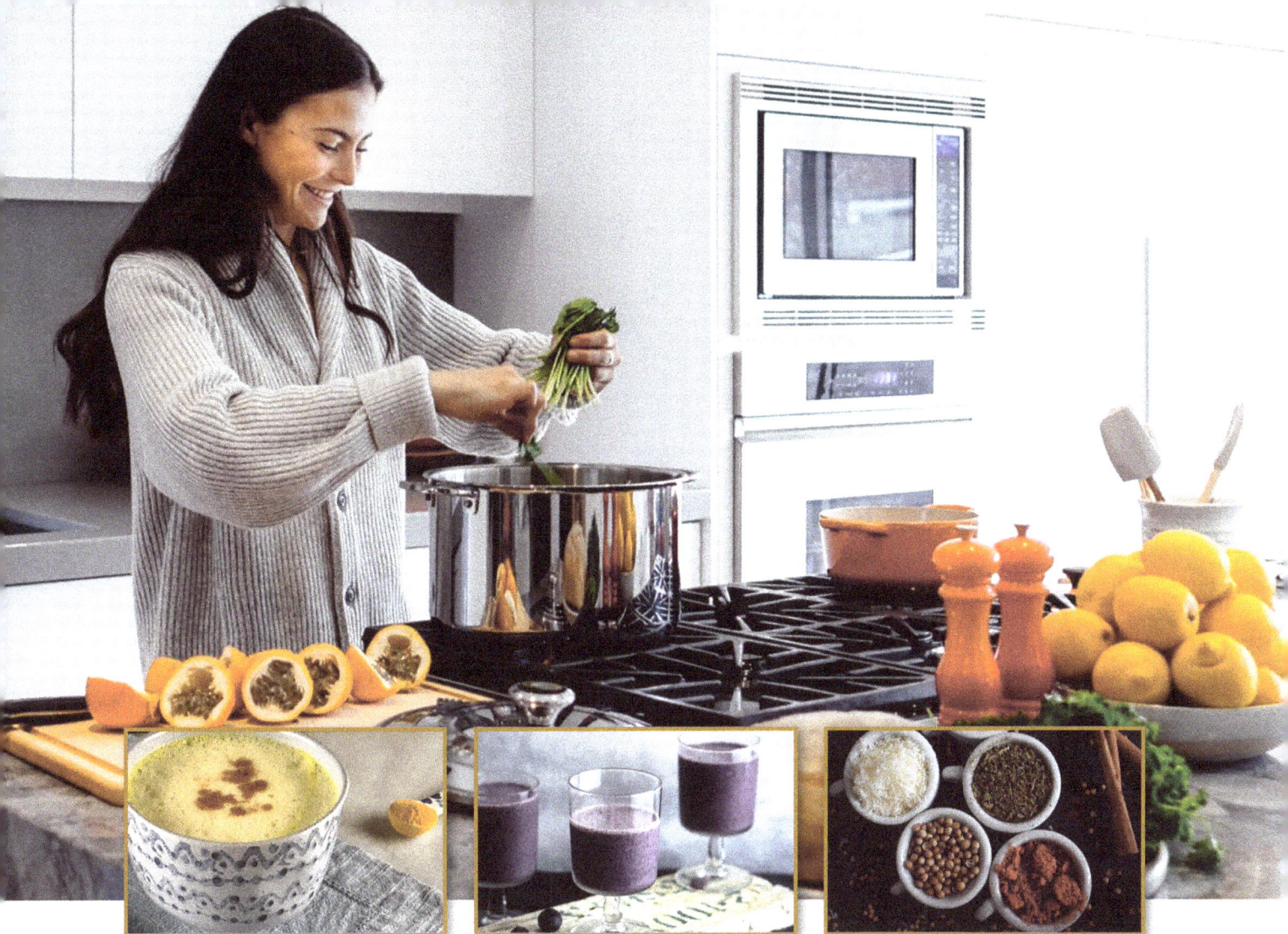

Cumin

Cumin is also packed with antioxidants and has also been shown to improve digestive system health. This helps the immune system by flushing out toxins and keeping your body in regular working order.

1. **Cumin baked chicken thighs.** Combine 2 tsp of cumin powder, 4 tbsp of olive oil, salt, pepper and 2 tsp of garlic powder. Rub over 4 chicken thighs and bake in the oven for 30–40 minutes until the skin is crisp and the meat is cooked all the way through.

2. **Coconut dahl.** Fry off one chopped onion, 1 tsp cumin seeds, 2 crushed garlic cloves, salt, pepper and 2 tsp masala powder. After a couple of minutes, add 2 tins of washed and drained lentils. Add two tins of coconut milk and simmer for 1 hour. When thick, add in a handful of fresh spinach to finish.

3. **Cumin crusted salmon.** Combine 2 tsp cumin powder, 2 tsp garlic powder, seasoning, 1 egg and almond meal/flour. Pack on the skin side of the salmon. Place on a baking tray and grill on medium heat for 15–20 minutes until cooked all the way through.

Cayenne Pepper

You might have seen cayenne mentioned in 'diet shots' or for 'fat burning' drinks. Well, it can actually do so much more for your body than just alleged 'fat burning'. Cayenne activates your circulatory system, increasing blood flow and the speed of immune cells getting transported around the body.

1. **Spicy cauliflower mash.** Steam a whole cauliflower until soft to touch. Use a hand blender to mix with 50g of butter, a teaspoon of cayenne and salt.

2. **Mango smoothie.** Blend 1 ½ cups frozen mango, 3 tablespoons greek yoghurt, ¼ teaspoon cayenne, ice, a little honey and your milk of choice. Blend until smooth.

3. **Sweet and spicy meatballs.** In a bowl, mix with your hands to combine 500g of mince (pork, beef or lamb works well), 1 egg, salt and pepper. Roll up into small balls and bake in the oven on a baking tray for 30 mins on medium heat or until cooked through. Meanwhile, combine a little orange juice, 1 tsp cayenne, 1 tbsp honey and 2 tbsp soy sauce. Use this to glaze the meatballs with once cooked.

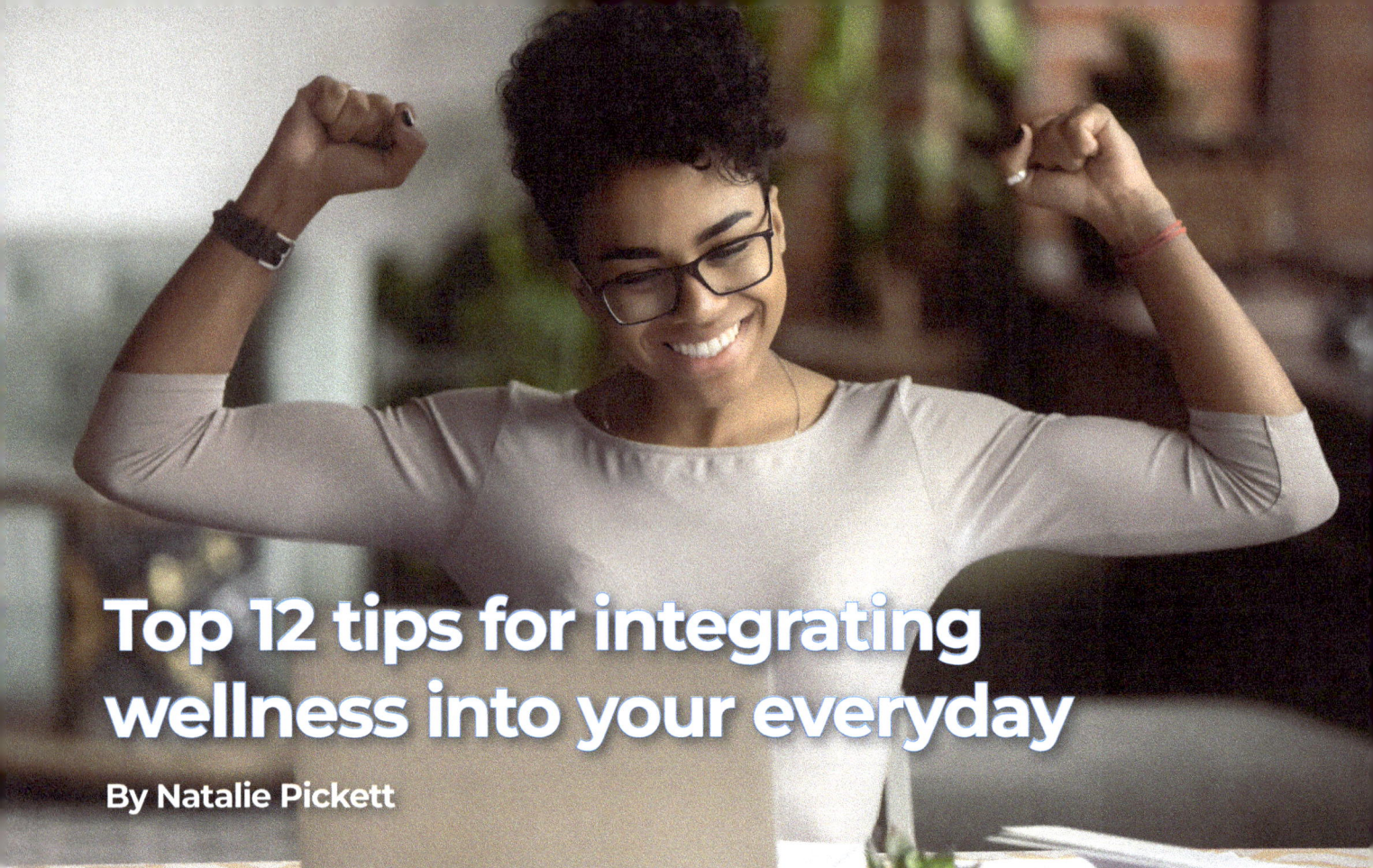

Top 12 tips for integrating wellness into your everyday

By Natalie Pickett

I've always been pretty active and have enjoyed exercising. This is one of the reasons why I turned that passion into my work by becoming a Fitness Instructor in the late 80s/early 90s (yes there was a lot of pink lycra involved too!).

My passion for fitness combined with my passion for travel as I worked my way travelling the east coast of Australia, then the USA and then onto the UK. This is where I crossed over to the travel industry, working for a European travel company, taking tours through Europe, before eventually settling back home in Melbourne, Australia and starting my own inbound travel company to showcase Australia to the world.

I appreciate that although I am passionate about keeping active, like many people, once my work became office-based and there is lots of work to do and lots of deadlines that don't involve you being physically active, it's easy to stop exercising and develop habits that are not so healthy. There's just too little time and we choose not make it a priority. 'I want to go to the gym, but this report is due and if I don't get if finished it will cause trouble!' Sound familiar? Once I had my daughter, I found it even harder to find time for me.

So how do we integrate wellness into our everyday activity?

In the speaking and business mentoring work that I do now, I present workshops on 'Goal Setting', where I talk about our patterns, how strong they are, and how they may be preventing us from achieving our goals. Is what we are doing now getting us closer to our goals? If not, we need to change what we are doing. If that change involves changing habits, it needs commitment, as it is very easy to slip back into old behaviours. We can easily step back into what we already know, even though those habits may not be taking us where we would like to go.

> We all have reasons why we don't move our bodies (aka exercise), and the most common reason for not finding ways to move throughout the day is 'time'.

In designing the program for 'Wellness on Time', I wanted to make sure that we made it easy, simple and fun for people to use and to integrate into their daily routine.

In doing so, I used examples from my own experience, feedback from others, and further research on creating new habits. We all have reasons why we don't move our bodies (aka exercise), and the most common reason for not finding ways to move throughout the day is 'time'.

Here are my 12 tips for integrating wellness into your everyday!

1   **Make it a priority.** Say it to yourself, say it to others – 'My Health and Wellness is Important to me!'

2   **Plan – saying it is one thing but action is key – do something about it!** Put it in your diary and make it a priority. By that I mean wherever possible not conceding that time for other appointments – put your wellness needs first.

3   **Don't try to do it all at once.** If the changes are too severe, you may find it difficult to keep it up. So rather than trying to change your whole lifestyle overnight, start with a small change and integrate that first.

4   **You don't have to be perfect.** Nothing can make you feel like quitting more than when you turn up for a group workout and you're struggling and everyone else seem to be a master at it! It is not a competition with others, it is about you improving, and has nothing to do with anyone else. Make small steps to improve your technique or efforts each time.

5   **Don't beat yourself up if you miss it.** If your goal was to include 3 x 30 minute workouts a week and you missed one, don't beat yourself up. Too much abstinence from the routine may cause you to feel like you're starting all over again and may cause you to feel like you're struggling to achieve your results. So yes, if you miss one, try and make it up. If not, just move on and make sure you make the next one.

6   **Be your own best friend.** This one is so important for wellness in life in so many ways. Watch your self-talk. Comments like calling yourself a 'loser' will most likely make you feel worse, and can have a negative effect in so many ways. Be your own support person. Acknowledge that you are improving, even if it is only small steps or by just turning up. A very wise healer once told me 'that little voice inside you should say the things to you that you would want your very best friend to say'. Be kind to yourself always.

7   **Feeling good.** It's not about the end goal. Changing to achieve healthy habits is not an end goal or an event, as your life is ever evolving. It is a process, a lifestyle choice. If you make changing the habit the goal, then what will you do when you reach your ideal weight, achieve however many reps, eat fruit and veg, feel good every day? You might stop. So embrace the process and enjoy the activities that you do, so that enjoyment and the benefits of feeling good as you make improvements becomes the reward, not the end goal.

8   **Get started today.** Small steps can make a big difference, we can so easily find reasons as to why we don't start today ... too busy, too tired, need new workout gear, and so on. Take a small step to get started today.

9   **Be specific.** Many of us may have done this in stating a new commitment or maybe a new year's resolution – making a statement like 'I will exercise more'. Instead try something like, 'I will do a minimum 3 x 30 minute walks/ workouts each week'. If you do more, that's great! Start with something that is not too constrictive so that you don't feel like dropping out straight away, but something that you can measure to say 'Yes! I did that this week!' Put it in your diary so you can fit it into your weekly schedule. If you miss one, make sure you get the next one.

10   **Repeat.** The more you do to make it part of your routine, the more likely you will make it instinctive and turn it into a habit. After a while you may find that if you skipped your workout you really miss it, and you will naturally adjust your schedule to fit it in elsewhere to make it up.

11   **What do I do if I need to take a break or a holiday?** Many of us start a new fitness routine when we know we have a holiday or vacation coming up. The thought of fitting into a swim suit after winter can be a bit daunting! So we ramp up the activity before we go and then it is easy to let all of your good work slip when you're away – but you don't need to. You may choose to include some of your regular activities but think of all of the holiday activities you can do whilst away that will keep you moving, snorkelling, stand-up paddle boarding, walks on the beach, hiking, cycling, sea kayaking, walking and bike tours. Make it fun! If your break from routine was due to illness or injury, consult with your health practitioner if needed to see what you can still do whilst injured, because you may need to adapt your program. For whatever reason you take a break, try and resume as soon as possible.

12   **Replace a not so good habit with a better one.** There is a lot of opinion around that says that it takes 21–30 days to break a habit or form a new one. From my research, I've discovered that whilst that may be true for some, this is based on an opinion published in a book in the 1960s and has been perpetuated as fact in a range of theories since. Although it seems that this is based on opinion rather than a scientific study, it is a good estimate. From what I've read and from my experience, changing a habit can be based on a range of factors, and can take anywhere between a few days to several months or even years.

Retreat (verb)

To 'retreat' is the act of moving back or withdrawing. Time spent away from one's normal life for the purpose of reconnecting in a quiet or secluded place in which one can rest and relax.

Re-treat
Re-charge
Re-store
Re-vive
Re-energise
Re-vitalise

Where is your favourite place for a retreat?

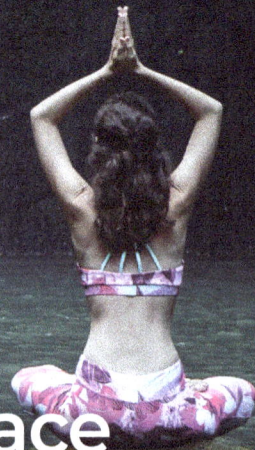

The healing power of pets

By Jane Thornton

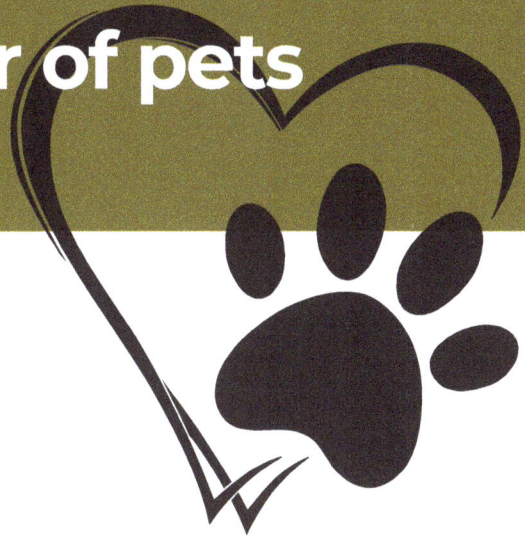

I have had pets my entire adult life – until recently. Possum, my darling tortoise shell, she shadowed me wherever I went. Rum Tug, the Burmese, he left too soon. Charlie, my first black and white Border Collie (BC) – when nothing else mattered, he single handedly taught me to keep an open heart. Taj, the white Siamese cross who found me, and Minette Cha, the black and white moggy, were my companions for eighteen years. Taj was my familiar – he knew and felt everything about me. Minnie puss, well, she was just always there.

Meg was my next BC, a unique blonde border collie. When I sat in the whelping pen, this little gold bundle crawled up my leg, tucked under my skirt and fell asleep. I was her chosen one and so the bond began.

Meggy Moo gave me gifts that are simply immeasurable. If one could have a furry soul mate, she was mine. We were in simpatico, inseparable, and simply in love. Fortune, fate, and fatality brought her brother, Gryff, to me for the last five years of their lives – they were two peas in a pod and had been since birth. It was pure joy to see them together, sleeping, playing, running, swimming, chilling out and how much they mirrored each other, and me. We were family, nay, they were my family, I didn't have children, but they were mine and we were blessed to have a small extended family that supported us when needed.

I'm in my 60s now, and Meg and Gryff passed two years ago close to each other. I miss them dearly, but memorialising them in portraits has created a healing, not only for myself, but a gift that I feel blessed to share. And so, I started Momento Pet Portraits in honour of my fur family.

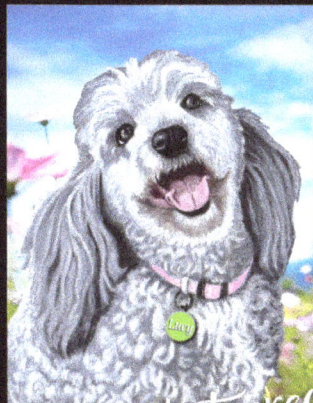

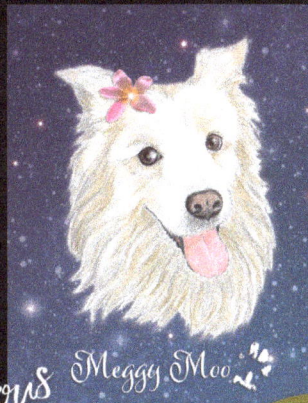

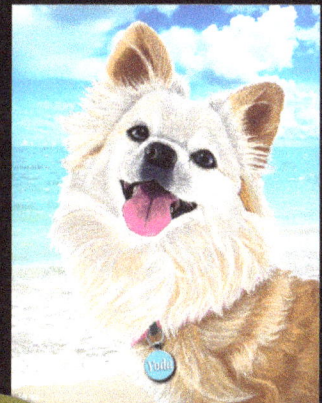

Book reviews

The Dictionary of Lost Words by Pip Williams
Affirm Press, 2020. Review by Caz.

At first glance, this novel is a charming tale of a child who, with a little bit of naughtiness and some level of bravery, collects words that have been rejected by the compilers of the first edition of the *Oxford English Dictionary* – words that have slipped through the cracks literally and metaphorically.

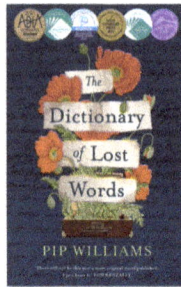

Wrapped around and throughout this tale is her journey through childhood. Her father is one of those responsible for the collection and selection of words for the dictionary. Her mother has passed away, and with no one to care for her after school, the dictionary compilers become her 'family'. Consequently, she often spends time at her father's workplace, sitting quietly and often unnoticed. Her secret collection of unwanted words become her treasures that she stores in a chest under her bed.

As her life proceeds, a suite of prejudices, assumptions and challenges emerge that mirror those prevalent for young women in the early 20th century. Her godmother, her education and her fascination with life in other parts of society add another level of engagement.

Words, however, are the true protagonist in this novel. They have the power to define truth and the capacity to represent and express our humanity. Pip Williams has created a fresh perspective on the value and the provenance of words. I read this book in one sitting. Then I read it again. I was, and remain, totally charmed.

The Bookbinder of Jericho by Pip Williams
Affirm Press, 2023. Review by Caz.

In the preface to this novel, Pip Williams introduces Peggy Jones, the bindery girl wearing a brown cotton-drill skirt and a wash-worn blouse. This preface is titled 'Before', and over six and a half pages, totally captivated me. Within this section, the mystery involved in the creation of a book, its journey though typesetting, printing, page folding, binding and even the leather book cover with the gold lettering of the titles, all contribute to the evocation of the romance of book making.

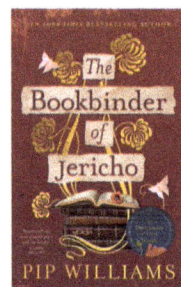

From there, the novel unfolds with Peggy the narrator and the Oxford University Press the central location. The novel is structured into five sections – each given the title of a book that Peggy helps to bind. The time stretches between the months prior to the outbreak of World War 1 to the end of the war in November 1918.

Peggy's identical twin sister Maude, their aunt Tylda, Jericho staff, Belgian refugees, Oxford university students and people living alongside Peggy and Maude on the canal, populate the novel and are the instruments of the themes of war, loss, love, hardship and hope. The dreams and aspirations of young women at this point in history resonate throughout the novel and accentuate the great gulf between the different social levels in the British class system. But the war caused the greatest opportunity for working class women to move out of gender restricted roles. Between them, Peggy and Maude represent opposite levels of ambition regarding work and social mobility. Will they maintain their close interdependence as they move past the time of war and into their adult lives?

Available for purchase from Readings https://www.readings.com.au

How to Keep House While Drowning: A Gentle Approach to Cleaning and Organizing
by KC Davis LPC
S&S/Simon Element, 2022
Review by Kellie Fowle, B Well Counseling

Attention-deficit/hyperactivity disorder (ADHD) is by far the most common diagnosis I work with. It comes with an array of challenges, with one being physical disorganisation. Your space has to make sense, or else it is so overwhelming that it can cause you to emotionally shut down. *How to Keep House While Drowning: A Gentle Approach to Cleaning and Organizing* is by far one of my favourite books to help organise the space you live in, and/or help those who live with you who have ADHD.

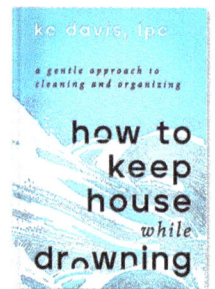

This is recommended for anyone who feels overwhelmed by their environment and feels like they are constantly cleaning up with no end result … freezing because there feels like there is too much to do, as if the busyness of life has left you to drown in the mess of your home. The author is a psychotherapist and a mum, and she struggles with executive dysfunction, so she is incredible at being able to normalise what so many of us feel, and offer real and tangible strategies on how to tackle the overwhelm. She also has worksheets and exercises on her website you can use to complement the book.

You can find the book here: https://amzn.to/3Vh12cg

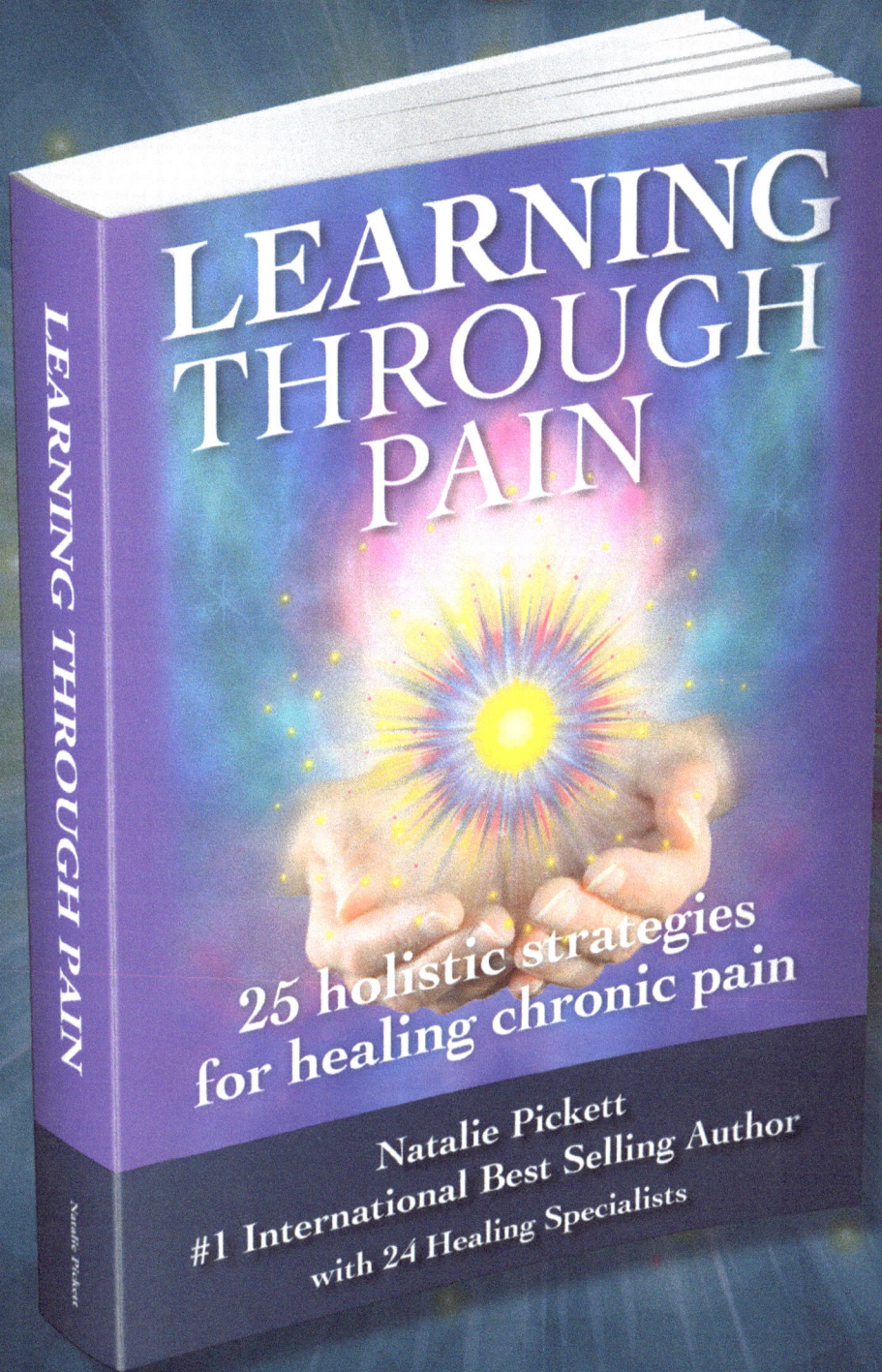

Word cloud word play

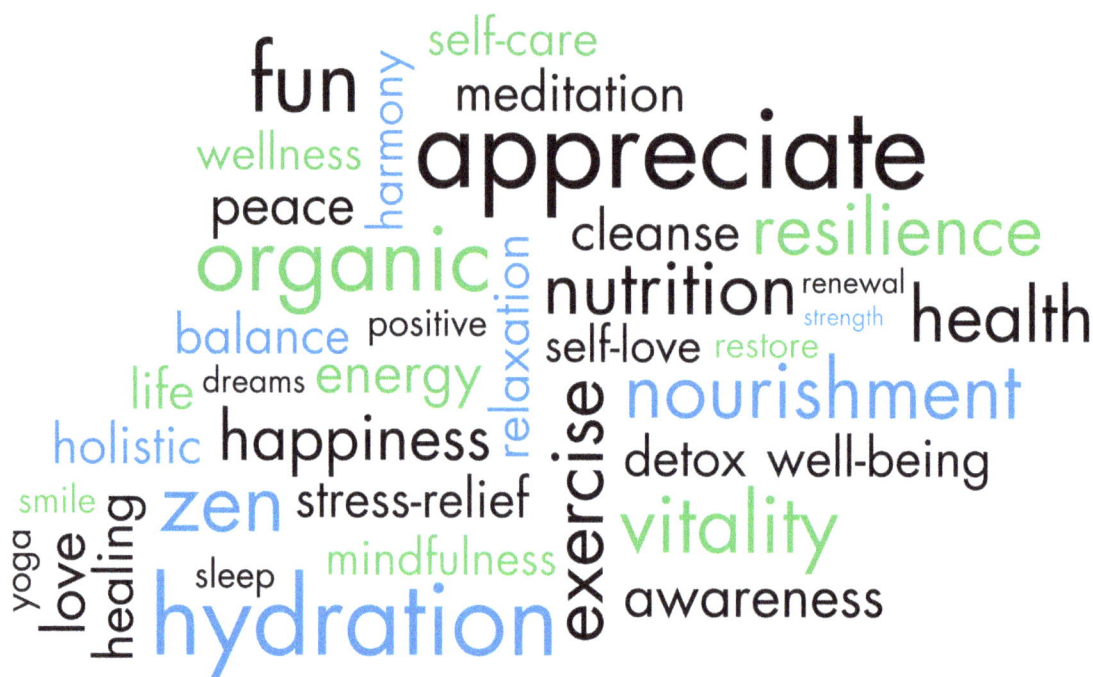

fun
harmony
self-care
meditation
wellness
appreciate
peace
cleanse
resilience
organic
nutrition
renewal
strength
health
balance
positive
self-love
restore
life
dreams
energy
relaxation
nourishment
holistic
happiness
exercise
detox
well-being
smile
zen
stress-relief
vitality
yoga
love
healing
sleep
mindfulness
awareness
hydration

Relax and take a minute to be mindful of your breathing. Take a few gentle deep breaths. Look at the word cloud. What words stand out for you? Any particular words that resonate? Write them below:

My words for today/week/month are:

What are the feelings that come up for me around these words?

Is this something that I want more of in my life?

What decisions and actions can I make to have more of this in my day?

Write your intentions for how you will integrate more of these activities in your day/week/month

www.ingramcontent.com/pod-product-compliance
Lightning Source LLC
Chambersburg PA
CBHW040926050426
42334CB00061B/3480